Marrow and Stem Cell Processing for Transplantation

Marrow and Stem Cell Processing for Transplantation

Editors

Larry C. Lasky, MD
Director, Division of Transfusion Medicine
Associate Professor of Pathology and Internal Medicine
Ohio State University College of Medicine
Columbus, Ohio

Phyllis I. Warkentin, MD
Director, Transfusion Services and Cell Processing Laboratory
Professor of Pathology and and Pediatrics
University of Nebraska Medical Center
Omaha, Nebraska

American Association of Blood Banks
Bethesda, Maryland
1995

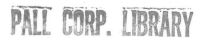

American Association of Blood Banks
8101 Glenbrook Road
Bethesda, Maryland 20814-2749

ISBN NO. 1-56395-042-1
Printed in the United States

Library of Congress Cataloging-in-Publication Data

Stem cell and marrow processing for transplantation/editors,
Larry C. Lasky, Phyllis I. Warkentin.
p. cm.
Includes bibliographical references and index.
ISBN 1-56395-042-1 (case bound)
1. Bone marrow—Transplantation—Congresses. 2. Haematopoietic stem
cells—Transplantation—Congresses. I. Lasky, Larry C. II. Warkentin, Phyllis I.
[DNLM: 1. Bone Marrow Transplantation—congresses. 2. Stem Cells—cytology—congresses. 3. Stem Cells—transplantation—congresses. 4. Bone Marrow—cytology—congresses. WH 380 S824 1994]
RD123.5.S74 1995
617.4′4—dc20
DNLM/DLC
for Library of Congress
94-47071
CIP

Contents

Foreword

This book is the result of a conference sponsored by the American Association of Blood Banks in Tampa, Florida, March 7-9, 1993. Approximately 250 people at all levels of expertise in marrow processing attended. The conference consisted of a series of presentations given by expert practitioners in marrow processing, followed by a question-and-answer panel discussion. Each presentation included introductory material; a review of the current knowledge, methods and practice; and a description of cutting-edge developments in the area under discussion.

Outlines of the talks were circulated among the speakers before the conference, not to minimize overlap, but to maximize it, and to ensure that each relevant area was discussed at least once. These outlines were made available to the attendees so that they could take notes during the conference. The outlines, taking into account the remarks of attendees and fellow speakers from the extensive discussion periods during the conference, were used to produce the chapters contained in this book.

Throughout this book, we have attempted to use uniform terminology. The term *progenitor cell* is used to mean a cell that can differentiate into daughter cells. A *stem cell* is a progenitor cell that is also capable of self-renewal. The phrase *peripheral blood stem cells* is used to denote a collection of leukocytes from the circulation that contains committed progenitor cells and, presumably, stem cells, as well as numerous other white cells. Autologous "transplant" is used to describe marrow rescue from high-dose chemoradiotherapy using the patient's own progenitor cells, derived either from the bone marrow or from the peripheral blood.

In our summary of the conference, we conceptually divided the presentations and, thus, the chapters in this book, into three categories. The first is the most basic, most important material, the quality control section. Gary Spitzer discussed using in-vitro progenitor cell assays for quality control and Janice Davis presented microbial quality issues.

In the next category are the issues we termed "bread and butter," the major procedures commonly performed in a cell processing laboratory. Charles Carter discussed automated methods for marrow processing, Patrick Stiff covered cryopreservation and Adrian Gee, Kenneth Anderson and Scott Rowley presented various aspects of purging autologous marrow of malignant cells. Nancy Collins discussed T-cell depletion of allogeneic bone marrow by various methods. Peripheral blood stem cells were also discussed.

The third category includes more investigative procedures and future applications. In each of these areas, preliminary studies of potential clinical applications are under way, but they have yet to be generally instituted in a large number of centers, or to be of proven utility or efficacy. These presentations included those by Hal Broxmeyer on cord blood stem cells, Shelly Heimfeld on the in-vitro expansion of hematopoietic progenitors and Irwin Bernstein on positive selection of progenitor and stem cells.

The conference and this resulting book were a production of the American Association of Blood Banks' Transplantation Immunology Committee, chaired during most of the planning and until the last few months before the conference by James Mason, PhD. There was input from all committee members, especially Barbara Gorgone. Scott Rowley, although not a member of the committee, was extremely instrumental in planning the conference and choosing the speakers.

Several AABB staff members at the National Office provided assistance toward our endeavor. Angela Buscemi and Helen Bishop, PhD, were key in planning the conference and David Singleton and Deanna Hines helped carry out the details of the conference. Carolinda Hales and Janet McGrath were responsible for publication of this book.

Larry C. Lasky, MD
Phyllis I. Warkentin, MD
Editors

In: Lasky L and Warkentin P, eds. *Marrow and Stem Cell Processing for Transplantation*
Bethesda, MD: American Association of Blood Banks, 1995

1

Clinical Background for Marrow and Progenitor Cell Processing

Phyllis I. Warkentin, MD

HEMATOPOIETIC STEM CELL TRANSPLANTATION is a potentially curative therapy for a variety of life-threatening diseases originating in or involving the bone marrow. These diseases include severe combined immunodeficiency disease (SCID), Wiskott-Aldrich syndrome, other immune deficiency or white blood cell disorders; acquired severe aplastic anemia, Fanconi anemia, inherited metabolic disorders such as the mucopolysaccharidoses, adrenoleukodystrophy and other storage diseases, and osteopetrosis; red cell disorders including thalassemia and selected cases of sickle cell anemia; and various malignant diseases of bone marrow such as acute leukemia, chronic myelogenous leukemia, myelodysplastic/myeloproliferative disorders, lymphoma and selected solid tumors of both children and adults, including neuroblastoma, Wilms' tumor, breast cancer and others.[1-15] Initially, almost all marrow transplants were performed using fresh anticoagulated marrow, obtained from a donor matched at the major histocompatibility complex (MHC) and manipulated as little as possible.[16,17] Since these successes, the identification of associated complications, especially graft-vs-host disease (GVHD) and recurrent leukemia; the observation that ABO compatibility was not required for successful transplant outcome; and improvements in the technology of hematopoietic cell cryopreservation, progressively more

---

Phyllis I. Warkentin, MD, Professor, Pathology and Pediatrics, and Director, Transfusion Service and Cell Processing Laboratory, University of Nebraska Medical Center, Omaha, Nebraska
(This work was supported by Transfusion Medicine Academic Award K07-HL0234-1 from the National Institutes of Health.)

1

precise laboratory methods of in-vitro bone marrow and peripheral blood progenitor cell processing have been developed.[18-23] The purposes of this chapter are to review the rationale, process, potential donors and clinical indications for hematopoietic stem and/or progenitor cell transplantation and to provide an introduction to hematopoietic progenitor cell processing and cryopreservation methodologies.

Rationale for Hematopoietic Stem Cell Transplantation

Bone marrow transplantation is utilized as definitive or adjuvant therapy for those patients with otherwise life-threatening diseases. Specifically, the purposes of marrow transplantation are: 1) to replace deficient or defective marrow cells with normal (donor) cells and 2) to restore normal hematopoiesis following high-dose or myeloablative doses of chemotherapy and/or radiotherapy. To achieve complete lymphohematopoietic reconstitution following marrow infusion, a preparative regimen is required. The purposes of the preparative regimen are: 1) to provide sufficient immunosuppression to allow the engraftment of allogeneic marrow and to avoid graft rejection and 2) to eradicate the underlying malignancy. The ideal preparative regimen would accomplish these purposes without unacceptable toxicity to the graft recipient. Combinations of high-dose chemotherapy with or without radiation therapy are given during the 4-12 days preceding the marrow infusion. Because of their antitumor effect and/or relative lack of toxicity, various preparative regimens have been developed by different transplant teams to treat different diseases.

Types of Transplants

Bone marrow transplantation is commonly divided into three categories based on the source of the donor cells.

Allogeneic transplant is the infusion of a bone marrow graft from an individual other than the patient or an identical twin; ie, a graft that is genetically nonidentical to the host. Data from the most recent survey by the International Bone Marrow Transplant Registry (IBMTR) representing 14,745 allogeneic bone marrow transplants performed in 342 institutions indicate that 83% of allogeneic transplants performed between 1988 and 1990 were done to treat a malignant disease.[14] Of the total transplant recipients, 47% had acute leukemia; 26% had chronic myelogenous leukemia; 5% had lymphoma; and 5% had another malignancy. Considerable data exist to suggest that the antitumor effect of allogeneic transplant is derived from both the chemoradiotherapy preparative regimen and an immune component, usually referred to as the graft-vs-leukemia effect.[24] Seventeen percent of the allogeneic transplants reported to the IBMTR were performed to treat nonmalignant diseases. Aplastic anemia accounted for 9% of the total transplants; 2.3% were for thalassemia major, 2.6% for immune deficiency and 1.7% for genetic metabolic disorders.[14] Allogeneic donors were related to the recipient in 92% of these transplants; they were usually siblings matched at the MHC. Eight percent of the donors were unrelated volunteers. Since only 25-30% of patients who could benefit from allogeneic bone marrow transplantation are likely to have a completely matched sibling donor, it is expected that unrelated donors will provide an increasing percentage of allogeneic bone marrow transplants in the future, aided by increases in the number and diversity of potential donors listed in the National Marrow Donor Program (NMDP). In contrast to these data, statistics from the NMDP demonstrate that approximately 43% of transplants performed using unrelated donor marrow are for chronic myelogenous leukemia; 34% are used to treat acute leukemia. Presumably, the length of time required for the donor search process, in part, accounts for the differing percentages, since patients with chronic leukemia are more likely to remain in stable condition during a donor search and to reach transplant.

Syngeneic transplant is the use of bone marrow from an identical twin. Theoretically, a syngeneic transplant could be used to treat any condition treated by allogeneic or autologous transplant, except those genetic diseases that would affect both twins. IBMTR data suggest that less than 2% of all nonautologous transplants are syngeneic.[14]

Autologous transplant is the infusion of previously stored normal bone marrow (or peripheral blood progenitor cells) from the patient to restore hematopoietic function following intensive chemotherapy and/or radiation therapy intended to cure a malignant disorder. Situations in which an autologous transplant may be considered should meet the following criteria: 1) a poor prognosis malignancy with minimal chance of cure using conventional therapy, demonstrably more sensitive to high-dose therapy than to conventional dose therapy; 2) the existence of effective cytoreductive therapy that has bone marrow suppression as its dose-limiting toxicity; and 3) the availability of a source of stem cells that is or can be rendered free of tumor. The ideal time for autologous transplant is when there is minimal tumor burden and the tumor is sensitive to therapy.[12] Diseases treated with autologous transplant include lymphoma; solid tumors such as neuroblastoma, Wilms' tumor, breast cancer, brain tumors and others; and leukemia.

Bone Marrow Collection

Regardless of the type of transplant being performed, the process of marrow collection is the same.[16,25] Bone marrow is collected under standard sterile conditions in an operating room. General or spinal anesthesia is required. The collection is usually from both posterior iliac crests using multiple punctures of the bone with large-bore needles designed specifically for marrow harvest. If it is necessary to obtain a suitable number of nucleated cells, marrow may also be obtained from the anterior iliac crests or, rarely, from the sternum. Small aliquots are removed and mixed immediately in anticoagulant, usually heparin with tissue culture media. Some transplant teams have used saline or other solutions approved for human infusion as diluents in the operating room, without apparent deleterious effect.[26] Aliquots of marrow are pooled into a beaker or semiclosed system,[27] and then filtered through 500- to 200-micron filters or stainless steel screens into a plastic blood bag. The marrow collection may then be infused directly or processed as indicated.

The target number of nucleated cells may vary, depending on the clinical situation; however, it is usual to collect at least 2×10^8 nucleated cells/kg of recipient body weight for allogeneic transplant and at least 1×10^8 nucleated cells/kg for autologous infusion. These amounts can usually be achieved by the collection of 10-20 mL/kg of recipient body weight. Much more marrow may be needed if the marrow is intended to be purged of potential malignant cells or T cells. These procedures usually require the harvesting of $4\text{-}6 \times 10^8$ nucleated cells/kg of recipient weight. The hematocrit of the harvested marrow is generally 0.25-0.35 (25-35%).

Both the age of the donor and the amount of prior chemotherapy may influence the concentration of nucleated cells in harvested marrow. There is suggestive evidence that marrow from very young children has a higher concentration of nucleated cells and probably of marrow repopulating cells than does marrow from adult donors. Thus, if a child donor is significantly smaller than the intended recipient, it is feasible to collect less volume and still achieve hematopoietic reconstitution in the recipient.[28]

Processing of Allogeneic Bone Marrow

Allogeneic bone marrow is usually infused fresh from the donor on the day of collection. Although successful cryopreservation of allogeneic marrow has been reported, it is not commonly practiced.[29] There are three principal reasons for which allogeneic bone marrow may be processed: 1) avoidance of hemolysis at the time of marrow graft infusion due to ABO incompatibility between donor and recipient by removal of mature red cells and/or plasma; 2) volume reduction in fluid-sensitive patients by removal of plasma; 3) avoidance of GVHD in the recipient by T-cell depletion.

ABO Incompatibility

ABO identity between bone marrow donor and recipient is not essential for the successful outcome of the transplant. The rate of marrow engraftment, incidence of rejection, incidence and severity of GVHD and patient survival have all been shown to be unrelated to the compatibility between donor and recipient for antigens of the ABH group.[19,20,30-32] These clinical observations, in addition to in-vitro experiments, have been interpreted to demonstrate the absence of ABH antigens on the pluripotent and very early committed stem cells in humans.[31,32] There may, however, be some significant immunohematologic consequences that can be avoided.[33]

Transplantation across ABO groups may involve the presence of antibody in the recipient directed against donor red cells (major incompatibility) or antibody in the donor against recipient red cells (minor incompatibility). In major ABO incompatibility, two immunohematologic complications are important: 1) the risk of severe hemolytic transfusion reaction at the time of the marrow infusion and 2) delayed erythropoiesis and/or persistent hemolysis following transplantation due to continued presence or production of the isohemagglutinins anti-A and/or anti-B by the recipient. Delayed erythropoiesis is commonly observed, regardless of the manner of patient preparation or marrow processing. Laboratory evidence includes a decrease in the percentage of early erythroid cells in bone marrow samples obtained on day 28 posttransplant, a significantly greater number of days to achieve a peripheral blood reticulocyte count >1%, and an increase in the number of red blood cell transfusions required by recipients of major ABO-incompatible marrow as compared to recipients of ABO-identical marrow infusions.[31] In minor ABO incompatibility, immune hemolysis at the time of marrow infusion as a result of passive transfer of isohemagglutinins in the plasma-containing marrow may occur, or delayed immune hemolysis caused by red cell antibodies produced transiently by the donor marrow lymphocytes could develop. Several methods have been described that successfully manage these potential complications.

Major ABO Incompatibility

Acute hemolysis as an immediate result of the infusion of ABO-incompatible bone marrow containing a large volume of mature red blood cells can be avoided either by in-vivo removal of the circulating isohemagglutinins from the recipient or by in-vitro removal of the mature red blood cells from the marrow inoculum prior to infusion. Both methods have been shown to be very effective.

Removal of circulating anti-A and/or anti-B from the recipient requires that large-volume plasma exchange be performed after the administration of immunosuppressive drugs and before the marrow infusion. Plasma exchange of twice the patient's estimated blood volume, repeated as necessary depending on initial and follow-up anti-A and/or anti-B titers, is most commonly recommended. In most patients, this results in a significant decrease in the circulating titer of isohemagglutinin.[19,20,30,34] The goal is to reduce the isohemagglutinin titers to <16. Some transplant teams have supplemented plasma exchange with in-vivo immunoadsorption of antibody by pretransplant infusion of donor-type red cells or purified A or B substance. These infusions have generally been well tolerated; however, the change in titer could not be predicted by the volume of cells infused.[20]

The major disadvantages of plasma exchange for isohemagglutinin titer reduction are related to the risks and potential complications of plasma exchange. Large catheters are required for the procedures. The central lines utilized for the remainder of the transplant are often unsatisfactory for maintaining the necessary blood flow rates. Simultaneous venous access is also needed for antibiotics and other supportive care measures in bone marrow transplantation. The replacement fluid utilized in the plasma exchange usually includes fresh frozen plasma (FFP) of the donor ABO group. FFP is associated with risks of allergic or other transfusion reaction and of transfusion-transmitted disease. There is a significant risk of bleeding, due to concomitant thrombocytopenia, and a risk of infection, due to the leukopenia produced by the chemoradiotherapy preparative regimen just completed. In addition, the relevant anti-A and/or anti-B titer may not fall as anticipated, and there may be reequilibration of both IgG and, to a lesser extent, IgM from the extravascular space, resulting in a rebound increase in antibody titer.[35]

As an alternative to isohemagglutinin removal, several methods have been reported by which to successfully remove mature red cells from the marrow inoculum. In the author's laboratory, a method was developed to deplete red cells in vitro from bone marrow before infusion using hydroxyethyl starch sedimentation in inverted plastic blood bags.[31] In the first 23 bone marrow samples processed using this technique, a mean of 97.8% of the red cells was removed with retention of 86.8% of the nucleated cells and 98.2% of the in-vitro granulocyte-macrophage colony-forming units (CFU-GM). The marrow inoculum infused contained a mean of 4.1 mL and a median of 2.7 mL of red cells (range, 0.4-21.8 mL). All patients had significant titers of both IgG and IgM isohemagglutinins before marrow infusion. All infusions were well tolerated. Despite the very small volume of red cells infused, laboratory evidence of transient hemolysis, including increased plasma hemoglobin, indirect hyperbilirubinemia and decreased serum haptoglobin, could be detected in some patients. These recipients of red-cell-depleted marrow grafts demonstrated bone marrow engraftment at the same rate as did recipients of ABO-identical or minor ABO-incompatible marrow.[31] Advantages of this method of in-vitro red cell depletion of marrow are that it is relatively easy to perform, is efficient for processing large volumes of marrow and is performed in a semiclosed system of blood bags. This method does not require the use of fetal calf serum or the expense of cell separator equipment. Compared to the single-step hydroxyethyl starch sedimentation procedure,[36] this method resulted in the recovery of a higher percentage of nucleated cells and CFU-GM, in the infusion of a smaller volume of incompatible red cells to the patients, and in a lower transfusion reaction rate at the time of the marrow infusion.

Various methods of in-vitro red cell depletion utilizing automated blood cell separators, with or without density gradient, have also been described.[37-43] Each of the techniques and blood cell separators has been successful, although the precise characteristics of the marrow grafts obtained and results reported are variable. It is important to consider the relative advantages and disadvantages of each technique and piece of equipment within the context of the specific intention for the graft and purpose of the processing. The following are examples of results obtained using some of the various automated blood cell separators.

The Fenwal CS-3000 automated blood cell separator (Baxter Healthcare Corporation, Deerfield, IL), using the routine lymphocytapheresis program, the Granulo separation chamber and the A-35 collection chamber, has been used without a density gradient solution to produce a nucleated cell concentrate largely depleted of mature red cells that is satisfactory for transplantation.[37,38] As described by Areman et al,[37] the procedure was designed to require minimal time and manipulation, to yield plasma suitable for use in further processing, and to yield red cells suitable for transfusion to the marrow donor, using only solutions approved for in-vivo administration. Bone marrow from 36 donors was processed by this automated technique. The average recovery of nucleated cells was 29.3%; that of mononuclear cells was 53.2%; of CFU-GM, 76.2%; and of red cells, 8.8 mL (range, 2.0-32.0 mL). Marrow graft recipients demonstrated engraftment that was comparable to that in patients receiving unmanipulated grafts; however, no data are presented that describe the infusion of the seven ABO-incompatible grafts.[37] Schanz and Gmür[38] processed 40 bone marrow samples using similar equipment and achieved 53.2% recovery of nucleated cells and 69.1% recovery of mononuclear cells with 4.0 ± 2.4 mL (range, 2-57 mL) of mature red cells. This series included three recipients of major ABO-incompatible allogeneic marrow grafts containing 19.2-27 mL of incompatible red cells. Two of these three patients experienced transient fever during the infusion of incompatible red cells. Thirty-nine of the 40 marrow donors received 311 ± 96 mL of recovered autologous red cells without complication.[38]

The COBE 2991 automated cell washer (COBE BCT, Lakewood, CO) has been used with Ficoll density gradient to process marrow for allogeneic recipients with major ABO-incompatible donors.[39] The resulting mononuclear cell concentrate contained a mean of only 1.17% of the original red cells, and all marrow infusions were well tolerated by the recipient. Two of the eight patients demonstrated reduction in serum haptoglobin after the infusion. There were no other reported manifestations of hemolysis or acute reaction.[39]

Table 1-1 illustrates the comparative results obtained by Preti et al[40] using either the Haemonetics V50 cell separator (Haemonetics Corporation, Braintree, MA) or the COBE 2991 cell washer without density gradient solution. Both methods produced mononuclear cell enrichment; however, the volume of red cells in the final product was quite high, particularly if they had been intended for infusion to ABO-incompatible recipients.

Pediatric bone marrow transplant recipients present unique challenges in marrow graft processing. Because the recipients vary from small infants to adolescents of adult size, the volume of marrow to process is also variable. The inefficiency of automated marrow processing of very small volume grafts has been reported by Saarinen et al.[41] In that study, 54 marrow samples from children weighing 7-65 kg were depleted of red cells with the Haemonetics V50. Marrow volumes ranged from 230-1145 mL, with 17 small (200-399 mL), 18 intermediate (400-799 mL)

Table 1-1. Bone Marrow Processing: COBE 2991 and Haemonetics V50[40]

	% Recovery	
	2991 (n=12)	V50 (n=12)
Volume	14 ± 1.3	11 ± 0.9
Nucleated cells	81 ± 2.1	52 ± 4.4
Mononuclear cells	85 ± 4.0	87 ± 4.1
CFU-GM	83 ± 7.8	62 ± 7.6
Red blood cells	23 ± 1.8	6 ± 0.3

and 19 large (800-1200 mL) volumes. Red cell mass was reduced by a median of 82%; however, the reduction of the red cell mass was more efficient with increasing initial marrow volume. The median reduction in red cell mass was 63% in the small-volume marrow, 82% in the intermediate-volume marrow and 88% in the large-volume marrow. In addition to the poor red cell reduction in the small-volume marrow, another disadvantage of this system is the requirement to add third-party, irradiated leukocyte-reduced red cells to the processing to achieve acceptable nucleated cell recovery.[41] Although the recipients of these grafts will ultimately be exposed to many blood donors, additional donor exposures to facilitate processing seem unnecessary.

Minor ABO Incompatibility

Minor ABO blood group incompatibility exists when the bone marrow donor has circulating anti-A and/or anti-B directed against the red cells of the marrow recipient. Immediate hemolysis after a minor ABO-incompatible transplant is rare; however, processing of the marrow graft by simple centrifugation with supernatant fluid removal is recommended.[20,33,44] Useful techniques have been described.[45] Most cases of significant hemolysis following minor ABO-mismatched marrow grafts are delayed 6-18 days after the infusion. The risk of hemolysis appears to be increased in recipients of T-cell-depleted grafts, and in those treated with cyclosporine for prophylaxis of GVHD.[33] Posttransplant transfusion with red cells of the donor ABO group and with plasma and platelets of the recipient type is recommended to minimize the severity of hemolysis.[20,33,44]

Volume Reduction

The total volume of fluid infused to the graft recipient can be reduced without significant loss of progenitor cells by processing of the marrow graft prior to administration. Simple centrifugation with removal of the supernatant fluid, as is used in the management of minor ABO incompatibility, is recommended.[44,45] Volume reduction may be indicated for patients who are small or fluid-sensitive, or those with preexisting fluid overload, cardiac compromise or renal dysfunction.

Depletion of T Cells From Allogeneic Marrow

Acute and chronic GVHD continue to be major causes of morbidity and mortality after allogeneic bone marrow transplantation, despite many improvements in both the prevention and treatment of these complications. Among recipients of MHC-identical sibling marrow grafts, the incidence of significant GVHD is approximately 50%, with mortality attributed to GVHD or its complications occurring in 15%-25%.[46] Factors that appear to increase the risk of development of acute GVHD include at least the following: mismatch for antigens of the MHC, unrelated donor and older age of the recipient.[46,47] Sex mismatching and donor parity have also been associated with an increased risk of acute GVHD.[48]

GVHD is essentially an immunologic assault of the marrow graft cells on the tissues and organs of the recipient, manifested acutely as diarrhea, rash and liver dysfunction. Criteria for the development of GVHD are: 1) transplantation of a graft containing immunologically competent cells, 2) presence in the host of important transplantation antigens that appear foreign to the immunocompetent graft and 3) immune incompetence of the host to reject the graft.[48,49] Data from studies of both animals and humans demonstrate that T lymphocytes contained in the donor marrow inoculum proliferate and differentiate in vivo and produce, either directly or through secondary mechanisms, the signs and symptoms of acute GVHD.[47] Recipients of allogeneic marrow grafts routinely receive some sort of prophylactic regimen in an attempt to prevent or modify the development of acute GVHD. Many clinical trials have concentrated on prophylactic drug therapy to prevent GVHD.

Both animal and human trials have demonstrated that the removal of T lymphocytes from the marrow inoculum can prevent GVHD.[50] Despite this success, most clinical trials have failed to demonstrate a survival benefit for recipients of T-cell-depleted grafts, for several reasons.[51] These patients have a higher nonengraftment rate than do recipients of T-cell-replete marrow grafts. They also have a higher leukemic relapse rate than recipients of unmanipulated marrow, probably because of the loss of the graft-vs-leukemia effect that accompanies GVHD. Finally, other complications, most importantly lymphoproliferative disorders associated with Epstein-Barr virus infection, occur more commonly in recipients of T-cell-depleted grafts.

The limiting-dilution assay of Kernan et al[50] has been reported to correlate with development of GVHD. No patient who received less than 1×10^5 T cells/kg developed GVHD, while four of seven patients who received 1.8×10^5 to 4.4×10^5 T cells/kg developed mild skin GVHD. This assay estimates the number of T cells necessary to initiate clinically detectable GVHD in an HLA-identical host. Partial depletion of T lymphocytes has been proposed as a method to avoid the complications of T-cell depletion while maintaining the benefit of avoiding clinically significant acute GVHD. Data from this assay are useful in making such calculations.

Marrow as harvested for transplantation usually contains $1\text{-}2 \times 10^{10}$ nucleated cells with 10-15% mature T lymphocytes.[51] This results in approximately $1\text{-}2 \times 10^7$ T cells/kg of recipient body weight. A variety of physical and immunologic methods have been developed to remove these T cells, including monoclonal antibody-based methods, E-rosette depletion with or without soybean lectin agglutination and counter-flow elutriation. These are described in detail later in Chapter 9. In general, some purification of the harvested marrow is required before the use of these specific methods for T-cell depletion. The initial step may be preparation of a buffy coat or a mononuclear cell concentrate.

Processing of Autologous Bone Marrow

Autologous bone marrow is usually processed to obtain a concentrate of nucleated cells, or sometimes mononuclear cells, prior to cryopreservation. Autologous marrow may also be processed to a variable extent before in-vitro tumor cell purging.[22,52] The purging agents used and the conditions required dictate the type of processing as described in detail in Chapter 7.

Autologous bone marrow is usually cryopreserved for a variable period of days to years before infusion. The purpose of the cryopreservation is to maintain viable stem and progenitor cells that are capable of restoring hematopoiesis following high-dose chemoradiotherapy, which is usually administered over several days. Cryopreservation also permits the prophylactic storage of tumor-free marrow to be used months to years later if needed. Even when autologous transplantation is planned to follow immediately after the marrow harvest, the marrow inoculum is usually cryopreserved. Although some unavoidable loss of hematopoietic stem cells occurs with processing and cryopreservation, progressive cell loss during proper frozen storage is not apparent.[23] Cryopreservation is not absolutely required for autologous marrow transplantation; however, there is a progressive loss of hematopoietic stem and progenitor cells during nonfrozen storage. Liquid storage of autologous marrow at refrigerator temperatures (4 C) for 3-5 days has been reported to be successful as measured both in vitro and in vivo.[53,54] Practically, the use of noncryopreserved autologous marrow requires that the entire dose of chemoradiotherapy be administered and that active metabolites of the drugs used be cleared from the circulation within the 3- to 5-day period. Many preparative regimens are longer than 5 days.

Various processing and cryopreservation techniques have been described.[23] At a minimum, preparation of a nucleated cell concentrate (buffy coat) prior to cryopreservation is required. This achieves depletion of most of the mature red cells in the collected marrow and reduction in the total volume. Various manual methods and semiautomated apheresis or cell washing devices are available, as described above for use in ABO incompatibility.[19,20,23,31,36-43,55-57]

For several reasons, it is desirable to remove mature blood cells from the marrow before cryopreservation. First, these cells are not important in reconstituting hematopoiesis following high-dose therapy and are not optimally preserved by the methods and cryoprotectants utilized for cryopreservation of hematopoietic progenitor cells. Further, they may interfere with processing, freezing, thawing and/or administration of the marrow if clumping occurs because of the presence of these damaged cells. Cryopreserved bone marrow or peripheral blood progenitor cells are routinely thawed rapidly near the patient's bedside and infused fairly rapidly without further processing or the use of a filter. Rowley et al[23] have reported a 50% loss of cells when clumping occurred, and infusion through a standard blood administration set was required.

Second, the presence of damaged mature cells may contribute to the toxicity of the marrow infusion. In one report, autologous bone marrow was cryopreserved without depletion of any of the mature red cells or volume.[57] After infusion of frozen-thawed marrow, all patients developed gross hematuria. Three of 33 patients developed acute nonoliguric renal failure immediately after the infusion, manifested by sharp increases in serum creatinine. At autopsy, the renal histopathology in all three cases was typical of the acute renal failure associated with an acute hemolytic transfusion reaction. It is likely that the stromal elements from the damaged red cells contained in the infusate contributed to the renal failure observed.

Third, failure to remove mature cells and a portion of the supernatant plasma and tissue culture medium prior to cryopreservation results in a larger total volume to be frozen. This requires that a larger quantity of dimethyl sulfoxide (DMSO) be used as the cryoprotectant. The quantity of DMSO infused may also contribute to the toxicity of marrow graft infusion.

Several investigators have observed toxicity associated with the infusion of previously cryopreserved marrow.[58-60] Davis et al[58] observed a higher incidence of infusion-related complications among those patients who received buffy coat cells than among those who received the more highly purified, light-density mononuclear cells. The toxicities observed are detailed in Table 1-2. The total quantity of DMSO may also have contributed to the toxicities observed. Stroncek et al[59] observed more infusion reactions among patients receiving cryopreserved marrow than among those receiving fresh allogeneic marrow (Table 1-3). In both studies,[57,58] the rate of bacterial contamination was significant; however, concomitant bacteremia in the marrow graft recipients was rare. Similar toxicities were observed among patients given infusions of cryopreserved autologous peripheral blood progenitor cells.[60] Both a larger total volume of cells—and hence cryoprotectant—infused and a larger volume of damaged mature red cells strongly correlated with the greater number of toxicities observed.

Table 1-2. Toxicities of Cryopreserved Marrow Graft Infusions[58]

	Buffy Coat Cells (n=58)	Density Gradient (n=26)
Nausea, vomiting	23	5
Flushing	13	0
Abdominal cramps	10	0
Dyspnea, chest tightness	8	0
Diarrhea	4	0
Headache	0	1
No complaints	18	20
	$p<0.01$	
Cardiovascular changes	57	22

Table 1-3. Toxicities of Marrow Infusions[59]

	Cryopreserved (n=134)	Fresh (n=71)
Chills	31.3%	1.4%
Nausea	44.8%	14.1%
Emesis	23.9%	8.5%
Fever	17.9%	0
	$p < 0.05$	
Headaches	3.0%	2.8%
Dyspnea	3.0%	1.4%
Bacterial contamination	12.7%	15.8%

Summary

Bone marrow transplantation is potentially curative therapy for many patients with otherwise life-threatening illnesses. Several sources of normal hematopoietic progenitor cells exist that can successfully reconstitute hematopoiesis after high-dose chemoradiotherapy. Many of these collections of progenitor cells will require processing and/or cryopreservation prior to infusion to the recipient. Various methods and pieces of equipment are available for these laboratory procedures. It is essential for the optimal supportive care of the transplant recipient that these progenitor cells be carefully and properly handled to ensure prompt engraftment after infusion.

References

1. Gatti RA, Meuwissen HJ, Allen HD, Hong R, Good RA. Immunological reconstitution of sex-linked lymphopenic immunological deficiency. Lancet 1968;2:1366-9.
2. Bach FH, Albertini RJ, Joo P, et al. Bone marrow transplantation in a patient with the Wiskott-Aldrich syndrome. Lancet 1968;2:1364-6.
3. Storb R, Champlin RE. Bone marrow transplantation for severe aplastic anemia. Bone Marrow Transplant 1991;8:69-72.

4. Flowers MED, Doney KC, Storb R, et al. Marrow transplantation for Fanconi anemia with or without leukemic transformation: An update of the Seattle experience. Bone Marrow Transplant 1992;9:167-73.
5. Krivit W, Shapiro EG. Bone marrow transplantation for storage diseases. In: Desnick RJ, ed. Treatment of genetic diseases. New York: Churchill-Livingstone, 1991:203-21.
6. Coccia PF, Krivit W, Cervenka J, et al. Successful bone-marrow transplantation for infantile malignant osteopetrosis. N Engl J Med 1980;302:701-8.
7. Lucarelli G, Galimberti M, Polchi P, et al. Bone marrow transplantation in patients with thalassemia. N Engl J Med 1990;322:417-21.
8. Beutler E, Sullivan KM. Bone marrow transplantation for sickle cell disease. In: Forman SJ, Blume KG, Thomas ED, eds. Bone marrow transplantation. Boston: Blackwell Scientific Publications, 1994:840-8.
9. Forman SJ, Blume KG. Allogeneic bone marrow transplantation for acute leukemia. Hematol Oncol Clin North Am 1990;4:517-33.
10. Thomas ED, Clift RA. Indications for marrow transplantation in chronic myelogenous leukemia. Blood 1989; 73:861-4.
11. Appelbaum FA, Barrall J, Storb R, et al. Bone marrow transplantation for patients with myelodysplasia. Ann Intern Med 1990;112:590-7.
12. Philip T, Armitage JO, Spitzer G, et al. High-dose therapy and autologous bone marrow transplantation after failure of conventional chemotherapy in adults with intermediate-grade or high-grade non-Hodgkin's lymphoma. N Engl J Med 1987;316:1493-8.
13. Armitage JO, Bierman PJ, Vose JM, et al. Autologous bone marrow transplantation for patients with relapsed Hodgkin's disease. Am J Med 1991;91:605-11.
14. Bortin MM, Horowitz MM, Rimm AA. Increasing utilization of allogeneic bone marrow transplantation. Results of the 1988-1990 survey. Ann Intern Med 1992;116:505-12.
15. Yeager AM. Bone marrow transplantation in children. Pediatr Ann 1988;17:694-714.
16. Thomas ED, Storb R. Technique for human marrow grafting. Blood 1970;36:507-15.

17. Thomas ED, Storb R, Clift RA, et al. Bone-marrow transplantation (first of two parts). N Engl J Med 1975;292:832-43.
18. Thomas ED, Storb R, Clift RA, et al. Bone-marrow transplantation (second of two parts). N Engl J Med 1975;292:895-902.
19. Bensinger WI, Buckner CD, Thomas ED, Clift RA. ABO-incompatible marrow transplants. Transplantation 1982;33:427-9.
20. Lasky LC, Warkentin PI, Kersey JH, et al. Hemotherapy in patients undergoing blood group incompatible bone marrow transplantation. Transfusion 1983;23:277-85.
21. Champlin R. T-cell depletion to prevent graft-versus-host disease after bone marrow transplantation. Hematol Oncol Clin North Am 1990;4:687-98.
22. Rowley SD, Jones RJ, Piantadosi S, et al. Efficacy of ex vivo purging for autologous bone marrow transplantation in the treatment of acute nonlymphoblastic leukemia. Blood 1989;74:501-6.
23. Rowley SD. Hematopoietic stem cell cryopreservation: A review of current techniques. J Hematother 1992;1:233-50.
24. Horowitz MM, Gale RP, Sondel PM, et al. Graft-versus-leukemia reactions after bone marrow transplantation. Blood 1990;75:555-62.
25. Treleaven JG, Mehta J. Bone marrow and peripheral blood stem cell harvesting. J Hematother 1992;1:215-23.
26. Schepers KG, Davis JM, Noga SJ. Comparison of standard bone marrow (BM) collection media to FDA licensed solutions (abstract). Transfusion 1993;33(Suppl):69S.
27. Lin A, Carr T, Herzig R, et al. Evaluation of a disposable bone marrow collection and filtration kit (abstract). Transfusion 1987;27:526.
28. Buckner CD, Petersen FB, Bolonesi BA. Bone marrow donors. In: Forman SJ, Blume KG, Thomas ED, eds. Bone marrow transplantation. Boston: Blackwell Scientific Publications, 1994:259-69.
29. Lasky LC, VanBuren N, Weisdorf DJ, et al. Successful allogeneic cryopreserved marrow transplantation. Transfusion 1989;29:182-4.
30. Hershko D, Gale RP, Ho W, Fitchen J. ABH antigens and bone marrow transplantation. Br J Haematol 1980;44:65-73.

31. Warkentin PI, Hilden JM, Kersey JH, et al. Transplantation of major ABO-incompatible bone marrow depleted of red cells by hydroxyethyl starch. Vox Sang 1985;48:89-104.
32. Karhi KK, Andersson LC, Vuopio P, Gahmberg CG. Expression of blood group A antigens in human bone marrow cells. Blood 1981;57:147-51.
33. Klumpp TR. Immunohematologic complications of bone marrow transplantation. Bone Marrow Transplant 1991;8:159-70.
34. Berkman EM, Caplan S, Kim CS. ABO-incompatible bone marrow transplantation: Preparation by plasma exchange and in vivo antibody absorption. Transfusion 1978;18:504-8.
35. Warkentin PI, Yomtovian R, Hurd D, et al. Severe delayed hemolytic transfusion reaction complicating an ABO-incompatible bone marrow transplantation. Vox Sang 1983;45:40-7.
36. Dinsmore RE, Reich LM, Kapoor N, et al. ABH incompatible bone marrow transplantation: Removal of erythrocytes by starch sedimentation. Br J Haematol 1983;54:441-9.
37. Areman EM, Cullis H, Spitzer T, Sacher RA. Automated processing of human bone marrow can result in a population of mononuclear cells capable of achieving engraftment following transplantation. Transfusion 1991;31:724-30.
38. Schanz U, Gmür J. Rapid and automated processing of bone marrow grafts without Ficoll density gradient for transplantation of cryopreserved autologous or ABO-incompatible allogeneic bone marrow. Bone Marrow Transplant 1992;10:507-13.
39. Blacklock HA, Gilmore MJML, Prentice HG, et al. ABO-incompatible bone-marrow transplantation: Removal of red blood cells from donor marrow avoiding recipient antibody depletion. Lancet 1982;2:1061-4.
40. Preti RA, Ahmed T, Ayello J, et al. Hemopoietic stem cell processing: Comparison of progenitor cell recovery using the Cobe 2991 cell washer and the Haemonetics V50 apheresis system. Bone Marrow Transplant 1992;9:377-81.
41. Saarinen UM, Lähteenoja KM, Juvonen E. Bone marrow fractionation by the Haemonetics system: Reduction of red cell mass before marrow freezing, with special reference to pediatric marrow volumes. Vox Sang 1992;63:16-22.
42. Zingsem J, Zeiler T, Zimmermann R, et al. Bone marrow processing with the Fresenius AS 104: Initial results. J Hematother 1992;1:273-8.

43. Lyding J, Zander A, Rachell M, et al. Bone marrow concentration using the COBE Spectra. J Clin Apheresis 1990;5:156.
44. Warkentin PI. Transfusion of patients undergoing bone marrow transplantation. Hum Pathol 1983;14:261-6.
45. Wadsworth LD, Herd SL, Stanley CE. Unique aspects of marrow collection, processing and transplantation in pediatric patients. In: Sacher RA, AuBuchon JP, eds. Marrow transplantation: Practical and technical aspects of stem cell reconstitution. Bethesda, MD: American Association of Blood Banks, 1992:129-55.
46. Vogelsang GB, Hess AD, Santos GW. Acute graft-versus-host disease: Clinical characteristics in the cyclosporine era. Medicine 1988;67:163-74.
47. Kernan NA, Bartsch G, Ash RC, et al. Analysis of 462 transplantations from unrelated donors facilitated by the National Marrow Donor Program. N Engl J Med 1993;328:593-602.
48. Sullivan KM. Graft-versus-host disease. In: Forman SJ, Blume KG, Thomas ED, eds. Bone marrow transplantation. Boston: Blackwell Scientific Publications, 1994:339-62.
49. Billingham RE. The biology of graft-versus-host reactions. Harvey Lect 1966;62:21-78.
50. Kernan NA, Collins NH, Juliano L, et al. Clonable T lymphocytes in T cell-depleted bone marrow transplants correlate with development of graft-v-host disease. Blood 1986;68:770-3.
51. Thomas ED. Marrow transplantation for malignant diseases. J Clin Oncol 1983;1:517-31.
52. Rowley SD, Davis JM, Piantadosi S, et al. Density-gradient separation of autologous bone marrow grafts before *ex vivo* purging with 4-hydroperoxycyclophosphamide. Bone Marrow Transplant 1990;6:321-7.
53. Lasky LC, McCullough J, Zanjani ED. Liquid storage of unseparated human bone marrow. Evaluation of hematopoietic progenitors by clonal assay. Transfusion 1986;26:331-4.
54. Ahmed T, Wuest D, Ciavarella D, et al. Marrow storage techniques: A clinical comparison of refrigeration versus cryopreservation. Acta Haematol 1991;85:173-8.
55. Stiff PJ, Koester AR, Weidner MK, et al. Autologous bone marrow transplantation using unfractionated cells cryopre-

served in dimethylsulfoxide and hydroxyethyl starch without controlled-rate freezing. Blood 1987;70:974-8.

56. Letheby B, Jackson J, Greally J, et al. Comparison of two methods of bone marrow processing for autologous bone marrow transplantation. In: Worthington-White DA, Gee A, Gross S, eds. Advances in bone marrow purging and processing. New York: Wiley-Liss, 1992:345-51.

57. Smith DM, Weisenburger DD, Bierman P, et al. Acute renal failure associated with autologous bone marrow transplantation. Bone Marrow Transplant 1987;2:195-201.

58. Davis JM, Rowley SD, Braine HG, et al. Clinical toxicity of cryopreserved bone marrow graft infusion. Blood 1990;75:781-6.

59. Stroncek DF, Fautsch SK, Lasky LC, et al. Adverse reactions in patients transfused with cryopreserved marrow. Transfusion 1991;31:521-6.

60. Kessinger A, Schmit-Pokorny K, Smith D, Armitage J. Cryopreservation and infusion of autologous peripheral blood stem cells. Bone Marrow Transplant 1990;5(Suppl 1):25-7.

In: Lasky L and Warkentin P, eds. *Marrow and Stem Cell Processing for Transplantation*
Bethesda, MD: American Association of Blood Banks, 1995

2

Progenitor Assays, How Much and When?

Gary Spitzer, MD; Sulabha S. Kulkarni, PhD; Nancy Kronmueller, MS; and Douglas R. Adkins, MD

WHICH VARIABLE(S) SHOULD BE evaluated to predict the transplantation potential of hematopoietic cells depends on what are thought to be clinically significant engraftment endpoints. An engraftment variable of potential significance is the early recovery of neutrophils or platelets, which may be a temporary phenomenon, but which would protect the patient against early infection or bleeding complications. In this circumstance, one would need to assay cells with limited proliferative and rapid differentiation potential. To evaluate the potential for long-term maintenance of blood counts following transplantation, an assay for cells with prominent self-renewal potential is desirable. Ideally, one would wish to assess both types of cell populations present within a stem cell product.

With the increasing number of ex-vivo manipulations of bone marrow or blood cells and the variable amount of chemotherapy patients may have received prior to autologous collections, these two populations of cells within the hematopoietic system can be depleted to variable degrees. The hematopoietic system is composed of a hierarchy of cells that exhibit progressively less potential for replication or self-renewal as the true stem cell differentiates to multilineage progenitors, lineage-restricted pro-

---

Gary Spitzer, MD, Professor of Medicine and Director, Division of Bone Marrow Transplantation; Sulabha S. Kulkarni, PhD, Associate Professor, Division of Bone Marrow Transplantation; Nancy Kronmueller, MS, Clinical Supervisor, Division of Bone Marrow Transplantation; and Douglas R. Adkins, MD, Assistant Professor, Division of Bone Marrow Transplantation, Oncology and Hematology, Saint Louis University, St. Louis, Missouri

genitors and, eventually, fully differentiated cells (Fig 2-1). Hematopoietic progenitor cells are believed to be the progeny of a single cell, the pluripotent stem cell. The pluripotent stem cell is endowed with the ability to reproduce itself and differentiate along two major cell lineages that ultimately give rise to different, mature, functional blood cell types. The lymphoid lineage produces T and B lymphocytes. The myeloid lineage differentiates into committed myeloid and erythroid progenitor cells, leading eventually to mature granulocytes, erythrocytes, monocytes and platelets. Recently, however, the hematopoietic stem cell has also been shown to generate a third major lineage, mesenchymal cells.

Hematopoietic progenitor cell assays have been an essential part of human bone marrow processing and purging technology. In recent years, these cellular assays have also been used in establishing the parameters for collection and transplantation of peripheral blood stem cells (PBSCs). Several assays for measuring different progenitor cells are currently in use in research and in the clinic.

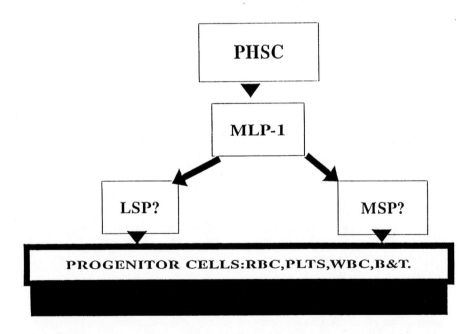

Figure 2-1. A subdivision of the hematopoietic system into different levels of differentiation. Most chemotherapy eliminates only the later parts of the system, the progenitor cells or preprogenitor cells. LSP = lymphoid stem cell; MSP = myeloid stem cell.

Assays in Semi-Solid Media

Progenitor assays are based on the ability of the various progenitor cells to produce in-vitro colonies in soft gel. The clonogenic cells are referred to as colony-forming units (CFUs), which are defined by the type of mature progeny that develops. Several in-vitro clonogenic test systems have been developed to measure CFUs for the various progenitor cell types.

The soft gels used in the progenitor assays are prepared from agar, methylcellulose or plasma clot. The marrow cells are suspended in the soft gel containing a nutrient culture medium, serum or plasma, and an appropriate colony-stimulating factor (CSF). During incubation at 37 C in humidified air containing 5-10% CO_2, the progenitor cells proliferate and differentiate to form cell colonies that are visible under an inverted microscope after 7-14 days in culture.

Blast colony-forming units (CFU-blast) are probably the earliest cell in the hierarchy of the differentiation scheme producing colonies, consisting exclusively of blasts, some of which are capable of producing secondary hematopoietic colonies upon replating. Proliferation and differentiation of marrow cells in CFU-blast culture are supported by early-acting hematopoietic growth factors. These colonies appear late in culture, at approximately 21 days. Another early colony-forming assay is high proliferative potential colony-forming cells (HPP-CFCs). These are colonies with significant replicating potential, which are generated after 21 days in culture that contains a mixture of early- and late-acting growth factors.

In the presence of appropriate CSFs, colony-forming unit—granulocyte/erythroid/monocyte/megakaryocyte (CFU-GEMM or CFU-MIX) produces colonies in soft gel consisting of granulocytes, erythrocytes, monocytes or macrophages and megakaryocytes. The human CFU-GEMM closely resembles the hematopoietic spleen colony-forming cell in the mouse. In addition to the CFU-GEMM, the differentiated progenitors that are committed to produce granulocytes and monocytes or macrophages (CFU-GM), erythroid cells [erythroid burst-forming unit (BFU-E) and CFU-E], and megakaryocytes (BFU-MEG and CFU-MEG) also form colonies in vitro. BFU-E and CFU-E represent the less and more mature forms, respectively, of committed erythroid progenitors, whereas BFU-MEG and CFU-MEG represent, respectively, the less and more committed megakaryocyte progenitors.

The CFU-GM assay is most frequently used clinically to evaluate stem cell preparations.

Liquid Culture Assays

Suspension culture, incorporating different growth factors with or without subsequent culture in semi-solid media, is increasingly being used as a useful alternative assay to provide additional information to the CFU-GM assay. With suspension cultures, proliferation can be determined by means of incorporation of ^{3}H-thymidine, and differentiation is determined by morphology and by flow cytometric immunophenotyping using a panel of monoclonal antibodies against myelomonocytic, erythroid and megakaryocytic antigens. A commonly used assay (Pre-CFU-C) to evaluate earlier cells than the CFU-GM involves treating the marrow or blood suspension with drugs such as cyclophosphamide, at doses that eliminate virtually all CFU-GM, and subsequently measuring the number of CFU-GM that differentiate from an earlier cell by sampling the liquid culture after 7 days.

A long-term bone marrow culture (LTBMC), referred to as the Dexter system, was developed for the production of marrow progenitors and some blood cells. The cultures were originally developed with murine bone marrow. Later modifications of this system were created for the growth of human cells. This system supports the proliferation and differentiation of pluripotent and committed progenitor cells for periods greater than 1 year for the mouse system and for shorter periods (4-6 weeks) for human bone marrow cells. In the long-term in-vitro culture system, proliferation of marrow cells is supported by an adherent layer of marrow stroma consisting of adipocytes, fibroblasts, endothelial cells and macrophages.

Limiting-dilution cultures of bone marrow or blood onto preformed stroma can provide a quantitative estimate of the cells responsible for the maintenance of these LTBMCs. The cells are referred to as long-term culture-initiating cells (LTC-ICs). Cells responsible for the maintenance of these cultures are considered the closest relative to the true hematopoietic stem cell that we can measure in vitro.

Application of Culture Systems

Both the soft-gel and LTBMC systems have been widely used in research and in the clinic. The semisolid system has been in use in the clinic as a quality control method for marrow processing and cryopreservation, used to ensure the viability and the repopulating capacity of the frozen marrow. This system is currently in use as a quality control method for hematopoietic progenitor cell concentration from bone marrow and peripheral blood. In research, it is used in the development of new marrow-purging protocols as a means of testing for potential hematopoietic toxicity of chemotherapeutic and immunotherapeutic purging agents. This method is valuable for assessing the cell kill after chemopurging with 4-hydroperoxycyclophosphamide (4-HC) alone or in combination with vincristine, as the cell number does not change significantly after such treatment. LTBMCs are also used to evaluate the effect of such treatments on multilineage myeloid stem cell survival. Despite the number of in-vitro assays available, only the CFU-GM, BFU-E, CFU-GEMM and indirect methods of evaluating the CFU-GM content of stem cell components (such as CD34 measurements) have been used to predict engraftment kinetics and to define the quality of the collection.

The Progenitor Cell Content of the Marrow Graft Predicts Engraftment Kinetics

Some of the questions raised concerning the use of evaluating CFU-GM in marrow transplantation are listed in Table 2-1. Spitzer and coworkers[1] investigated the potential for the CFU-GM assay to be predictive for hematopoietic recovery after high-dose therapy, and they were the first to report a correlation

Table 2-1. Questions About CFU-GM Use

- Is CFU-GM only valuable for identifying a threshold of stem cells required for hematopoietic engraftment?
- Does CFU-GM linearly relate to recovery of neutrophils?
- What are the numbers for ABMT?
- What are the numbers for PBSC?

between the number of committed hematopoietic progenitors infused during autologous transplant and the rapidity of hematopoietic recovery. In this study, patients who received a larger number of CFU-GM (as measured on day 10 of the progenitor assay) had a more rapid peripheral blood neutrophil recovery after high-dose therapy. Douay et al[2] also reported that recovery of CFU-GM predicted engraftment after autologous bone marrow transplantation (ABMT). However, several other investigators have found little or no correlation between the numbers of CFU-GM infused and hematopoietic recovery.

Roodman et al[3] investigated the utility of the CFU-GEMM assay for predicting hematologic recovery in patients with solid tumors uniformly treated with high-dose melphalan and cryopreserved autologous marrow rescue. They compared the value of CFU-GEMM assay to that of late (CFU-E) and early (BFU-E) erythroid progenitor assays in predicting hematologic recovery. Using multivariate analyses, they found that CFU-GEMM assays, but not CFU-E or BFU-E, predict both platelet and neutrophil recovery.

These studies indicate that both CFU-GM and CFU-GEMM assays may be used to determine the repopulating ability of cryopreserved bone marrow. Inadequate numbers of these progenitor cells (after freezing) are predictive for dangerously slow neutrophil recovery when marrow alone is used for transplantation.

How Much Is Enough for Autologous Bone Marrow Transplantation?

Spitzer et al,[1] examining hematopoietic recovery after high-dose therapy and ABMT given without growth factors, demonstrated that a minimal number of CFU-GM ($1-2 \times 10^4$/kg) were needed to ensure against prolonged, life-threatening neutropenia in patients receiving myeloablative therapy. There was a log-linear correlation between hematopoietic recovery and the dose of CFU-GM infused.

Douay et al[2] reported a lack of linear correlation between hematopoietic recovery and the dose of CFU-GM infused, but they also reported the existence of a CFU-GM threshold with respect to engraftment. Patients receiving doses of $>1 \times 10^3$ CFU-GM/kg had significantly faster hematopoietic recovery than patients receiving below this threshold value. The median day posttransplant of recovery to 0.5 and 1.0×10^9 neutrophils per liter in those patients receiving more or less than the threshold value of CFU-GM were on days 14 and 15 vs days 29 and 31.5 (p <0.05 and p <0.02), respectively; the median days to recovery to 1.0 and 2.5 × 10^9 leukocytes/liter were days 12.5 and 16 vs days 28 and 30.5 (p <0.05 and p <0.02), respectively. Considering the period of the first 4 weeks posttransplant, the authors showed that white blood cell recovery was significantly faster in the patients receiving doses of CFU-GM >1 × 10^3/kg (p <0.001). Correlations with the number of CFU-GM infused and hematopoietic recovery still hold true after treatment with drugs ex vivo.[4,5]

Sequential studies evaluating the reappearance of CFU-GM in the marrow and the peripheral blood after high-dose therapy and ABMT indicate that the in-vivo kinetics of CFU-GM recovery predict engraftment. By day 7 after transplantation, CFU-GM were already detectable in the marrow in patients with optimal engraftment, at a level of 10% of the dose infused. The detection of circulating CFU-GM in the blood by day 10 or day 14 was indicative of engraftment.[1,2]

Studies by Roodman et al[3] of engraftment kinetics revealed that transplantation of at least 35 × 10^3 CFU-GEMM/kg of body weight resulted in normal rate of recovery of neutrophils and platelets, but transplantation of <28 × 10^3 CFU-GEMM/kg resulted in delayed hematologic recovery.

Adequate viability of cryopreserved marrow stem cells is crucial to successful engraftment. A greater than 50% recovery of CFU-GM, after freezing, was shown to ensure engraftment in transplant patients. Analysis of these samples by CFU-GEMM assay and Dexter's LTBMC showed that the pluripotent stem cells, which are responsible for sustained engraftment, and CFU-GM behaved similarly after cryopreservation.

In summary, the CFU-GM progenitor cell assay predicts the rate of early neutrophil recovery after ABMT, without posttransplant growth factors. This is surprising, given the variations in the assay, in different operators, in pre- and postfreezing recoveries, etc. Although there is no absolute threshold of CFU-GM required for infusion after high-dose therapy, it would be important to infuse an adequate amount of CFU-GM that would be predictive for a reasonable duration of cytopenia. Recovery by day 28 after ABMT to 500 neutrophils/μL when growth factors are not used, and by day 21 after ABMT when growth factors are used would be considered worrisome extremes, and the infusion of at least the number of CFU-GM (2 × 10^4/kg before freezing) associated with this rate of neutrophil recovery would be prudent. With these recommendations, mortality related to infection would be anticipated to be reasonably low.

Although recommended doses of CFU-GM for rapid myeloid engraftment have been reported, it has been demonstrated that hemopoietic reconstitution following 4-HC-purged ABMT ultimately can occur even when the CFU-GM and the more primitive CFU-GEMM are not detectable within the marrow. However, recovery is slow, with a major proportion of these patients not realizing 500 neutrophils/μL until well after 28 days. Many do not recover adequate platelet numbers.[4,5] Although European investigators have aimed for a residual 5% CFU-GM after purging the marrow with mafosfamide, workers at Johns Hopkins have simply treated patients with a defined dose of 4-HC. Both groups have claimed satisfactory clinical long-term outcome that apparently justifies the increased early morbidity and mortality. Carlo-Stella et al[6] investigated the effect of mafosfamide at the level of CFU-blast and found that the concentrations of mafosfamide required to eliminate more primitive hematopoietic progenitor cells, such as the CFU-blast, were significantly higher than those required to eliminate CFU-GM.

These studies suggest that suboptimal numbers of more mature progenitors are predictive for slow neutrophil recovery and potential complications but are not predictive for absence of engraftment. Evaluation of more primitive progenitors would provide insight into the engraftment potential of a marrow depleted of mature progenitors. Assays of both primitive and mature progenitor cells would be valuable in determining an appropriate in-vitro dose of drug to purge leukemic bone marrow. It is unlikely that marrow or blood would be depleted of CFU-GM and still have abundant primitive progenitors except after in-vitro purging. Failure to generate CFU-GM in vivo would be an indirect measurement of inadequate primitive hematopoietic cells.

How Much Is Enough for Peripheral Blood Stem Cells?

The answer to this question is again dependent on the rate of hematopoietic recovery. For instance, if we accept the neutrophil recovery discussed above, Kessinger and others[7] have shown that the number of CFU-GM required for PBSCs is similar to the guidelines noted for ABMT. Infusing approximately 1×10^4 CFU-GM/kg is associated with the same kinetics of hematopoie-

Table 2-2. Relationship of CFU-GM in Peripheral Blood to Hematopoietic Recovery[9]

	CFU-GM > 11.6*	CFU-GM < 11.6
Neutrophils > 500/μL	12 (9-21)	19.5 (11-60)
Platelets > 50,000/μL	15 (9-45)	40 (8-120)

* × 10^4/kg

tic recovery as was observed with the use of ABMT.[7,8] Use of PBSCs has been associated with the expectation of faster neutrophil and platelet recovery. To achieve these more ambitious goals, a total of approximately 10 × 10^4 CFU-GM/kg (or more) is recommended from the studies of Reiffers et al[9] (Table 2-2). To et al[10] have reported that infusion of 50 × 10^4 CFU-GM/kg obtained from PBSCs will reliably produce rapid and sustained engraftment. This group reported that, while initial engraftment remains rapid with lower doses, a CFU-GM dose >50 × 10^4/kg is important for sustained hemopoietic recovery (Table 2-3). A decline in blood counts after initial hematopoietic recovery after PBSC infusions is dependent on both the myeloablative potential of the conditioning regimen used and the potential absence of more primitive progenitors within the PBSC component. Obviously, higher numbers of CFU-GM are generally predictive for larger numbers of primitive progenitor cells, but this relationship in the mobilized peripheral blood product is complicated, and different assays must be incorporated to measure this relationship adequately. For instance, these critical values of CFU-GM for predicting hematopoietic recovery after PBSC infusion have been estimates derived from using PBSCs collected upon the rapid upswing after chemotherapy, with or without growth factor. The same numbers may not necessarily apply with the use of PBSCs collected after several days' administration of subcutaneous granulocyte colony-stimulating factor (G-CSF) or granulocyte/macrophage colony-stimulating factor (GM-CSF). Such different clinical protocols will likely have different guidelines for adequate PBSC collections.

Table 2-3. Occurrence of Trough Platelets (<25 × 10^9/L)[10]

CFU-GM	Numbers With Trough	Steady State
<50 × 10^4/kg	3/3	1/3
>50 × 10^4/kg	4/11	11/11

Do CD34-Positive Cells Predict the CFU-GM Content of Peripheral Blood Stem Cells Adequately?

Surface antigens present on progenitor cells have been used for rapid evaluation of the quality of the PBSC product. Several investigators have noticed a modest linear correlation between the number of CFU-GM and CD34+ cells in PBSC collections. Siena et al[11] have reported in one patient poor engraftment with infusion of $<6 \times 10^6$ CD34+ cells/kg of body weight. Schwartzenberg et al[12] reported that an apheresis product with $>2.5 \times 10^6$ CD34+ cells/kg will usually contain $>20 \times 10^4$/kg of CFU-GM, an adequate number for rapid hematopoietic recovery. However, a number of other investigators have noted poor correlation between numbers of CD34+ cells and CFU-GM, when cells are collected after certain mobilization techniques. In addition, other investigators observed a poor correlation between CD34+ cell numbers and hematopoietic recovery.[13]

To evaluate if CD34+ cell number is predictive for both early and sustained neutrophil and platelet recovery after high-dose chemotherapy given with PBSC support (in which apheresis components were collected after recombinant growth factor administration), the authors analyzed hematologic recovery following high-dose therapy in 57 patients who underwent apheresis after receiving the combination of a late-acting growth factor (G-CSF) and an intermediate-acting growth factor (GM-CSF). GM-CSF and G-CSF doses were 2-5 µg/kg and 3-10 µg/kg, respectively, given for 6 days prior to apheresis and during a median of 5 days of collections. The preparative regimens were cyclophosphamide, etoposide and cisplatin; cyclophosphamide, BCNU and etoposide; and mitoxantrone and thiotepa. Beginning one day after the infusion of autologous marrow and PBSCs, patients received G-CSF at 15 µg/kg/day and GM-CSF at 3-6 µg/kg/day (both as 2-hour intravenous infusions twice a day) until absolute neutrophil count was

Table 2-4. Recovery After Growth-Factor-Mobilized PBSCs

ANC*			Platelets	
>100/µL	>500/µL	>1000/µL	>20,000/µL	>50,000/µL
9 (8-14)[†]	11 (8-27)[†]	11 (8-27)[†]	15 (6-137)[†]	17 (9-137)[†]

* = absolute neutrophil count
[†] = median (range)

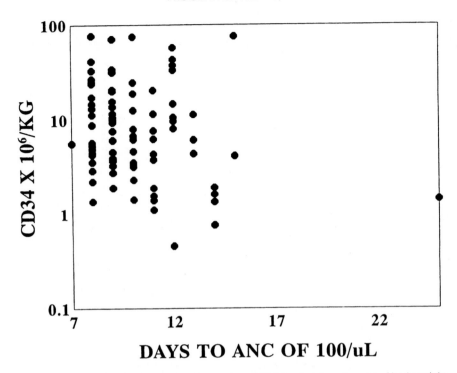

Figure 2-2. The relationship between the number of CD34 cells infused per kg of body weight and recovery of granulocytes after high-dose therapy and infusion of peripheral blood cells collected after growth factor infusion. Most patients received bone marrow as well. No significant relationship was discovered.

>1500/μL. Recovery of neutrophils and platelets with this approach was rapid, as shown in Table 2-4.

Several variables revelant to the hematopoietic response to growth factor before and during apheresis were examined to determine if any would be predictive for a high yield of CD34+ cells or CFU-GM in the PBSC collections. A high initial rise (day 1-5) of neutrophils and total white blood cells correlated with a high CD34+ cell apheresis yield, while early monocyte response correlated with high CFU-GM yield. However, the number of CD34+ cells infused did not correlate with rate of hematopoietic recovery (Fig 2-2 and 2-3). High white cell or absolute neutrophil counts during apheresis and continued administration of growth factors (days 7-15) are predictive for rapidity of neutrophil recovery after transplantation. In this study, the patient response to growth factor during apheresis collection is more predictive of early neutrophil recovery than is the number of CD34+ cells infused.

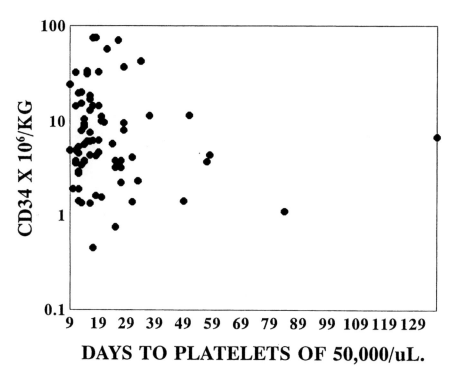

DAYS TO PLATELETS OF 50,000/uL.

Figure 2-3. The relationship between the number of CD34+ cells infused per kg of body weight and recovery of platelets after high-dose therapy and infusion of peripheral blood cells collected after growth factor infusion. Most patients received bone marrow as well. No significant relationship was discovered.

Conclusions

Late progenitor assays provide important information that can be used to exclude, on the basis of progenitor number below certain threshold guidelines, autologous bone marrow or peripheral blood cell collections that would be inadequate for yielding a

Table 2-5. CFU-GM Recommendations

ABMT Without Growth Factors

- If >500/μL granulocytes within 14 days are expected, collect >10 × 10⁴ CFU-GM/kg

ABMT With Growth Factors

- If >500/μL granulocytes within 14 days are expected, 1 × 10⁴ CFU-GM/kg may be adequate
- Growth factors make up for the extra progenitors that are responsible for the early differentiation into mature myeloid cells

Table 2-6. Relationship of CFU-GM in Peripheral Blood with Hematopoietic Recovery

CFU-GM per kg	Neutrophil Recovery	Platelet Recovery	Trough* Week 5 or 6
$>50 \times 10^4$	<14 days	<21 days	Some
$10\text{-}50 \times 10^4$	<14 days	<28 days	Frequent if ablative therapy used
$1\text{-}10 \times 10^4$	14-28 days	Median 4-7 weeks; may not occur	NR
$<1 \times 10^4$	>28 days	Frequently may not occur	NR

*More frequent if patient is heavily pretreated or has acute myelogenous leukemia.

reasonable period of hematopoietic recovery after high-dose therapy. Both late and early progenitor cell assays are important to evaluate after ex-vivo manipulations of stem cell components. The lack of agreement on the exact numbers of specific progenitor cells required relates to a combined lack of standardization of the assays and lack of understanding of all the growth factors needed for early and late hematopoietic recovery. Nevertheless, approximate recommendations can be made, depending on the desired rapidity of hematopoietic recovery. The components of hematopoietic recovery and a synthesis of the recommendations for the numbers of CFU-GM to be infused are provided in Tables 2-4 through 2-6.

References

1. Spitzer G, Verma D, Fisher R, et al. The myeloid progenitor cell—its value in predicting hematopoietic recovery after autologous bone marrow transplantation. Blood 1980;55:317-23.
2. Douay L, Gorin N, Mary J, et al. Recovery of CFU-GM from cryopreserved marrow and in-vivo evaluation after autologous bone marrow transplantation are predictive of engraftment. Exp Hematol 1986;14:358-65.
3. Roodman GD, LeMaistre CF, Clark GM, et al. CFU-GEMM correlate with neutrophil and platelet recovery in patients receiving autologous marrow transplantation after high-dose melphalan chemotherapy. Bone Marrow Transplant 1987;2:165-73.

4. Rowley SD, Zuelsdorf M, Braine HG, et al. CFU-GM content of bone marrow graft correlating with time to hematologic reconstitution following autologous bone marrow transplantation with 4-hydroperoxycyclophosphamide-purged bone marrow. Blood 1987;70:271-95.

5. Rowley SD, Piantadosi S, Santos GW. Correlation of hematologic recovery with CFU-GM content of autologous bone marrow grafts treated with 4-hydroperoxycyclophosphamide. Culture after cryopreservation. Bone Marrow Transplant 1989;4:553-8.

6. Carlo-Stella C, Mangoni L, Almici C, et al. Differential sensitivity of adherent CFU-blast, CFU-MIX, BFU-E, and CFU-GM to mafosfamide: Implications for adjusted dose purging in autologous bone marrow transplantation. Exp Hematol 1992;20:328-33.

7. Kessinger A, Armitage JO, Landmark JD, et al. Autologous peripheral hematopoietic stem cell transplantation restores hematopoietic function following marrow ablative therapy. Blood 1988;71:723-7.

8. Haas R, Ho AD, Bredthauer U, et al. Successful autologous transplantation of blood stem cells mobilized with recombinant human granulocyte-macrophage colony-stimulating factor. Exp Hematol 1990;18:94-8.

9. Reiffers J, Leverger G, Marit G, et al. Hematopoietic reconstitution after autologous blood stem cell transplantation. In: Gale RP, Champlin R, eds. Bone marrow transplantation: Current controversies. New York: Alan R. Liss, 1989:313-20.

10. To LB, Haylock D, Thorp D, et al. The optimization of collection of peripheral blood stem cells for autotransplantation in acute myeloid leukemia. Bone Marrow Transplant 1989;4:41-7.

11. Siena S, Bregni M, Brando B, et al. Circulation of CD34+ hematopoietic stem cells in the peripheral blood of high-dose cyclophosphamide-treated patients: Enhancement by intravenous recombinant human granulocyte-macrophage colony-stimulating factor. Blood 1989;74:1905-14.

12. Schwartzberg LS, Birch R, Hazelton B, et al. Peripheral blood stem cell mobilization by chemotherapy with and without recombinant human granulocyte colony-stimulating factor. J Hematother 1992;1:317-27.

13. Janssen WE, Farmelo MJ, Lee C, et al. The CD34+ cell fraction in bone marrow and blood is not universally predictive of CFU-GM. Exp Hematol 1992;20:528-30.

In: Lasky L and Warkentin P, eds. *Marrow and Stem Cell Processing for Transplantation*
Bethesda, MD: American Association of Blood Banks, 1995

3

Bacterial and Fungal Contamination of Stem Cell Components

Janice M. Davis, MAS, MT(ASCP)SBB

HEMATOPOIETIC STEM OR PROGENITOR cell transplantation is a therapy used to treat patients with a wide variety of malignant and nonmalignant diseases. Sources of hematopoietic cells include bone marrow, peripheral blood, cord blood and fetal liver. All of these components contain both committed and uncommitted progenitor cells. However, they are collected by different techniques, and they are distinct with regard to their cellular composition. All of the components, some more than others, are at risk of bacterial and fungal contamination during the collection procedure. Additional manipulations may increase the incidence of contamination. Reagents (eg, media, density-gradient solutions, deoxyribonuclease) that are routinely used during the processing procedures are not approved for injection by the Food and Drug Administration (FDA). Since patients may be cytopenic on the day of transplant and are often immunosuppressed, the infusion of a contaminated stem cell component may add to the morbidity and mortality of the transplant procedure. However, contamination does not mean that the cells should be discarded, because the stem or progenitor cell collections are unique and, depending on the situation, it may be impossible to replace them. Rather, it means that policies must be in place to address the infusion of culture-positive stem or progenitor cell components and that precautions must be taken to reduce the incidence of contamination.

Janice M. Davis, MAS, MT(ASCP)SBB, Technical Director, Cell Processing Laboratory, The Johns Hopkins Oncology Center, Baltimore, Maryland

Bacterial Contamination

Bone Marrow

There are three potential sources of contamination for bone marrow: the collection procedure, ex-vivo manipulations and bag breakage at the time of thawing and infusion (cryopreserved marrow only). Bone marrow cells are collected in the operating room with the donor-patient in the prone position so that the marrow can be aspirated from the posterior iliac crests.[1] Before aspiration, the skin is scrubbed from mid-thorax to mid-thigh with poloxamer-iodine solution, which is removed with sterile saline. The skin is punctured, and multiple bone punctures are made to obtain marrow. Bone marrow grafts were originally collected into open reusable beakers containing preservative-free heparin and tissue culture medium.[2] The mixture was then filtered through stainless steel screens to achieve a single-cell suspension. Some institutions continue to use this technique. In 1987, however, a disposable harvest kit was introduced that consists of a large funnel-shaped bag to which a series of closed filters can be attached.[3]

The open harvest system and percutaneous collection technique may introduce bacteria into the bone marrow component, but so may the tissue culture medium and anticoagulants. In 1986, one institution reported that three bone marrow harvests were found to be contaminated with *Pseudomonas putida*.[4] These bacteria were detected during routine surveillance cultures. Examination of the reagents used to collect the bone marrow revealed that the sodium heparin without preservatives was contaminated. Two of the marrow harvests had been infused before the results were known, and neither patient had clinical signs of bacteremia. However, antibiotic therapy was started within 24 hours of infusion.

Autologous and allogeneic bone marrow harvests are manipulated ex vivo. Autologous cells are concentrated,[5] cyropreserved[6] and, often, purged of contaminating tumor cells.[7] Allogeneic bone marrow harvests may be processed to remove erythrocytes,[8] plasma[9] and lymphocytes.[10] These techniques are varied, and the same result can be achieved with different procedures. Some of these procedures require that the cells be transferred to test tubes,[11] and others[12] use reagents not approved for injection by the FDA. These multiple steps in open systems compounded by often lengthy (8-12 hour) procedures may increase the incidence of contamination of the bone marrow aliquots.

A series of 100 bone marrow samples was monitored for bacterial contamination.[1] In this study the marrow was collected into open beakers. No antibiotics were added to the marrow at any time during the collection or processing. Seventeen percent of the marrow samples were culture-positive after collection. Buffy-coat concentrates were prepared from 37 of the 100 collections by the use of blood bags and a centrifuge before the cells were treated with 4-hydroperoxycyclophosphamide.[7] Four of the 37 became culture-positive after processing. These cells were thawed in a 37 C waterbath containing tap water. One thawed marrow sample was culture-positive, but not because of a ruptured bag. Bacterial monitoring was accomplished by inoculating 1 mL of bone marrow into a radiometric aerobic blood culture bottle containing tryptic soy broth and ^{14}C-labeled glucose. The bottles were incubated at 37 C and sampled for 7 days after which terminal subcultures were performed and held for 48 hours. All of the organisms were identified by standard biochemical assays.

In this series, all of the bacteria detected were organisms usually described as skin flora: *Staphylococcus epidermidis*, *Corynebacterium* species, *Bacillus* species, *Propionibacterium* species and *Streptococcus viridans*. The number of organisms in the samples was low, with contamination being detected on the average of 4 days after inoculation. No infectious complications could be ascribed to the marrow infusions. No patient who received culture-positive bone marrow had a positive blood culture containing the same organism within 7 days of infusion. In addition, there was no statistical difference in the incidence of fever in the patients who received culture-positive or culture-negative marrow. This study also included results from four experiments in which bone marrow samples were inoculated with *S. epidermidis* that had been isolated from a harvested bone marrow. Samples were maintained at 24 C and 37 C, and the level of contamination was determined over a 24-hour period. The bone marrow exhibited bactericidal properties, with the number of bacteria decreasing over time. It should be noted that these marrow samples were unmanipulated and, therefore, contained granulocytes. These same observations may not be seen if the bacteria were inoculated into a light-density cell fraction or another type of stem or progenitor cell component.

Schepers et al[13] reported a follow-up study of another 100 bone marrow harvests collected at the same institution. The follow-up was prompted by the following procedural changes: the use of the disposable harvest kit, the use of a cell washer to prepare a light-density cell fraction and the use of a different bag [the Fenwal Cryocyte Bag™ (Baxter Healthcare Corporation, Deerfield, IL)] for cell storage. Over 1200 of these bags have been thawed in this laboratory without a single break, as compared to a 1% incidence of rupture associated with the bags used in the first study (unpublished observation). The surveillance and microbiologic procedures were the same as in the first report. The incidence of contamination in the harvest samples decreased from 17% to 5%; contamination in the autologous postprocessing samples decreased from 11% to 2%. The organisms identified were skin flora, and there were no clinical complications associated with the infusions.

Lazarus et al[14] reported the incidence of contamination for 194 bone marrow harvests. These cells were collected into open beakers containing tissue culture medium and heparin. No antibiotics were added to the marrow or given to the marrow donors or recipients. Samples (0.1 mL) of bone marrow were inoculated onto blood, chocolate and anaerobic blood agar plates that were held for 48 hours in a 5% CO_2 incubator. Only one harvest sample was found to contain bacteria (*Moraxella* species and *Enterococcus* species). This contamination rate (1%) was much lower than the 17% seen in the earlier study using the same collection procedure. This difference may be related to the inability of this particular surveillance system to detect low numbers of bacteria, considering the length of time (48 hours) that the plates were examined and the median day (4 days) that the blood culture bottles became positive in the previous study. Of these 194 marrow samples, 175 were processed, 22 to remove erythrocytes due to ABO major blood group incompatibility and 153 to be cryopreserved for autologous infusion. None of the postprocessing samples were culture-positive. The cryopreserved autologous marrow was stored in a polyolefin bag and thawed in a waterbath containing sterile saline. Twelve of the 153 (8%) marrow samples were culture-positive after thawing. The predominant organisms were gram-negative bacilli (including five *Pseudomonas* species). In these 12 cases, seven of the bags ruptured during the thawing process. The authors suggested that the contamination occurred when the marrow came in contact with the waterbath; however, microbiologic testing of the material used in the thawing and storage of the marrow was negative. One patient experienced bacteremia; fever occurred within hours of infusion and blood cultures were positive for *P. picketti* and *P. paucimobilis*. These organisms were also isolated from the thawed marrow. Fortunately, the patient did respond to the antibacterial agents administered.

Stroncek et al[15] examined 134 autologous bone marrow harvests. In that series, antibiotics (penicillin and streptomycin) were added to 72% of the marrow samples during the procedure, but there was no difference in contamination rates based on the presence or absence of antibiotics. The marrows were thawed in a 37 C waterbath containing saline. Cultures taken at the time of infusion showed a 12.7% (17/134) incidence of contamination; however, seven of the 17 marrow samples were culture-positive before cryopreservation. Six of the marrow samples contained *Pseudomonas* species. Contamination was not associated with a particular processing or purging technique, nor with bag breakage in the waterbath. Again, no clinically significant problems were noted at the time of infusion.

Other Hematopoietic Stem or Progenitor Cells

The next most frequent source of hematopoietic cells for transplantation is peripheral blood. Autologous peripheral blood stem cell transplantation has been used to restore marrow function after high-dose therapy in patients with a variety of diseases. This approach has an advantage over bone marrow transplantation in that the patient avoids the risks of anesthesia associated with the collection of bone marrow. It also allows patients with an unaspirable bone marrow the option of high-dose therapy followed by autologous hematopoietic cell support. The progenitor cells are collected with the same apheresis devices that are used to prepare platelet concentrates and to perform therapeutic apheresis procedures, as described in Chapter 10.[16,17] Since these systems use disposable software and anticoagulants that are approved by the FDA for injection, one would expect that the incidence of bacterial contamination might be similar to that reported for apheresis platelets (1.6-3.2%).[18,19] However, contamination was not mentioned in any of the abstracts from the Second International Symposium on Peripheral Blood Stem Cell

Autografts.[20] This may be due to one of the following: 1) sterility quality control was not performed, 2) contamination was not detected or 3) the infusion of culture-positive products did not cause any clinical problems. Another potential source of contamination with this collection procedure is the needle puncture.[21] Bacteria can enter the blood component in the crypts and glands of a skin "core" cut out by the venipuncture site. Depending on the policy of the institution, vascular access may be achieved using venipuncture[16] or the use of a double-lumen central venous access device.[17] After collection, there is usually minimal manipulation of the peripheral blood stem cell component before cryopreservation. However, some investigators have used Ficoll-Hypaque to further fractionate the cells.[22] As with other cryopreserved components, there is a risk of contamination at the time of thawing, as a result of waterbath contamination and bag breakage.[23]

Cord blood has been shown to be an alternative to bone marrow as a source of transplantable stem or progenitor cells[24] and has been used to successfully transplant patients with Fanconi's anemia[25] and juvenile chronic myelogenous leukemia.[26] None of the authors reported contamination of the components, possibly because antibiotics were added to the cells after collection. However, the open system used to collect the cord blood is a potential source of contamination. The collection begins after the infant is delivered and the cord clamped.[27] The distal end of the cord is placed in a beaker containing acid-citrate-dextrose (ACD). The clamp is released and the blood flows into the beaker. Then penicillin and streptomycin are added to the mixture. Blood may also be removed from the placenta by using 20-gauge needles and syringes containing ACD. Early experiments have shown that manipulation of the cord blood cells resulted in large losses of progenitor cells,[24] so current techniques employ cryopreservation of the cells without manipulation.

Fetal liver cells in combination with fetal thymic cells have been used as a source of hematopoietic cells for patients who undergo transplantation to correct severe combined immunodeficiency disease (SCID) and a variety of congenital and hematologic disorders.[28] The same cells have also been used for in-utero transplantation of fetuses with SCID and thalassemia major.[29] The cells are prepared a few hours after fetal death. The liver and thymus are removed aseptically and processed with a homogenizer to prepare a single-cell suspension in tissue culture medium. For in-utero transplantation, the cells are injected into the umbilical vein under ultrasonic visualization. The authors stated that special attention was directed toward the prevention of contamination during the procedure.[29] However, the risk of contamination associated with the collection and processing of these cells is obvious.

Fungal Contamination

Fungal infections are a leading cause of morbidity and mortality after chemotherapy-induced neutropenia.[33] *Candida albicans* and *Candida tropicalis* infections have been the most common, with the second most frequent fungal infection being aspergillosis. Since aspergilli are ubiquitous fungi, stem or progenitor cell components can be contaminated during any open collection procedure or ex-vivo manipulation. Thus far, no series has been reported regarding the incidence of fungal contamination of stem or progenitor cell components. However, many laboratories have only recently begun to monitor these collections for fungal contamination.

Equipment as a Source of Contamination

As mentioned in the report by Lazarus et al,[14] bacterial contamination appeared to be associated with cells coming in contact with the environment when the bag ruptured in the waterbath during the thaw procedure. However, this could not be proven, since microbiologic testing of materials used in thawing and storing the marrow were negative. The authors postulated that the organisms could have been on the exterior surface of the freezing bags or metal plates, but samples obtained from the outside of vials and freezing bags were culture-negative. Most laboratories disinfect waterbaths with 10% bleach after each use. It is also good laboratory practice to dry the waterbath after cleaning so that organisms cannot survive in any residual water droplets.

A theoretical concern for components stored in liquid nitrogen is microbial cross-contamination. Some pathogens can maintain viability at low temperatures.[30] Viruses were stored in glass vials in a liquid nitrogen storage tank. Some of the vials broke, and samples of liquid nitrogen from the tank were examined. Infectious viral particles were detected, indicating the potential biohazard of liquid nitrogen storage. Blood components stored in liquid nitrogen could be considered at risk for cross-contamination if there were blood on the outside of one bag and a crack in another bag. To reduce this risk, Rowley and Byrne suggested the use of vapor-phase nitrogen storage.[31] However, the problem with vapor-phase storage is that there are wide temperature fluctuations inside the container when the unit is opened. A possible solution to this problem is the replacement of the standard steel frames with aluminum frames. This change in design reduces the temperature fluctuations and allows for vapor-phase storage. Another option for short-term storage of progenitor cells may be the use of the dimethylsulfoxide (DMSO)/hydroxyethyl starch method of cryopreservation[32] which uses a −80 C mechanical freezer. However, it MUST be remembered that cross-contamination of components stored in liquid nitrogen is a theoretical concern, and no illness has been attributed to marrow contamination during storage in liquid nitrogen.

Practical Considerations

Standards are currently written for monitoring hematopoietic stem and progenitor cell components for bacterial and fungal contamination. The American Association of Blood Banks *Standards*[34] states that "a representative sample of each bone marrow or peripheral blood progenitor cell harvest shall be tested for bacterial and fungal contamination after collection and processing. The medical director is responsible for review of the results."[34] The National Marrow Donor Program's most recent *Standards* state that every marrow must be placed into culture for bacteria and fungi at the transplant center, employing aerobic and anaerobic conditions.[35]

These standards are somewhat vague to allow for the fact that the science or art of stem or progenitor cell processing is continually evolving. These standards do not specify how to perform the microbiologic studies. An informal sampling of procedures employed by five transplant centers in the United States revealed varied practices. All of the laboratories used 0.5 to 1.0 mL of marrow sample for sterility testing. Three of the laboratories inoculated aerobic blood culture bottles. Two sampled the bottles for 7 days, with one performing terminal subcultures. The third group examined the bottles for 14 days. The fourth laboratory inoculated thioglycolate media and examined the media for 7 days, while the last laboratory inoculated blood and chocolate agar plates and thioglycolate media, examining them for 7 days. Fungal contamination was monitored by four of the five laboratories. Sabouraud dextrose agar slants were inoculated and examined for 14 (one laboratory) or 21 (three laboratories) days. One laboratory also used brain-heart infusion slants, which were examined for 21 days.

Guidelines for the Infusion of Culture-Positive Components

The procedures that should be followed when a hematopoietic stem or progenitor cell harvest is found to be culture-positive depend on when the laboratory is notified of the contamination in relation to the scheduled day of infusion. As mentioned above, there was only one reported clinically significant reaction associated with the infusion of a contaminated bone marrow. However, fatal septic reactions have been reported when immunocompromised patients were transfused with contaminated platelets,[36,37] so contamination should not be ignored or treated casually.

If the laboratory staff is informed that a stem or progenitor cell collection is culture-positive before the infusion (which can happen only when the component has been cryopreserved), the following events should occur. The laboratory medical director should be notified immediately, and the microbiology department should be made aware of the importance of identifying the organism(s) as well as determining sensitivities. The medical director is responsible for notifying the patient's attending physician. Notification will most likely depend on the type of organism isolated and the time required for the specimen to become positive after inoculation (an indirect measure of the level of contamination). However, decisions may have to be based on the results of only a Gram's stain. Antibiotics can be administered before and possibly after the infusion. When the culture-positive component is thawed, samples should be taken for sterility testing to determine if it was truly contaminated or if the sample was contaminated in the microbiology department. The bedside staff should be prepared for a septic transfusion reaction to the infusion. Septic transfusions are characterized by high fever, shock, disseminated intravascular coagulation and renal failure.[38] Other symptoms may include diarrhea, vomiting and general muscle pain. However, these other symptoms may be difficult to assess when the component has been cryopreserved, because they may be related to the infusion of DMSO and not to bacterial contamination.[39] Treatment of the symptoms includes the administration of intravenous antibiotics combined with therapy for shock.[38] Since bags of cryopreserved components are thawed sequentially, each bag should be infused and the patient should be stable before the next bag is thawed. This reduces the potential for clumping of the cells in a thawed component while the staff is waiting to infuse a medically unstable patient.

If the laboratory is notified of a culture-positive collection after the cells have been infused, the medical director should still be notified. Antibiotics may need to be administered depending on the organism(s) identified and the patient's medical condition.

Documentation

The laboratory should prepare a surveillance report on a monthly or quarterly basis to document the results of sterility testing for all components. The report should be reviewed by the medical director. When there is a culture-positive component, the microbiology department staff should document in their records that they have notified the responsible person concerning the contaminated blood component. Once the processing laboratory has been informed, documentation should begin with the medical director and his or her interaction with the patient's physician. This should be recorded in the patient's laboratory record and possibly in the patient's chart. Laboratory documentation for all culture-positive stem or progenitor cell components should include the following: the patient's maximum temperature and antibiotics administered on the day of infusion, any reaction to the infusion (eg, chills, changes in blood pressure) and blood culture reports within the first week after transplant. When the organism identified is not considered to be skin flora, more extensive documentation is necessary. The laboratory should have a copy of the following: the infusion record (which is part of the patient's chart and includes vital signs and the nursing notes recorded during and after the infusion), a list of antibiotics administered on the day of transplant and any other pertinent medical information such as physician notes and blood culture results. This information should be included in the Surveillance report prepared from the bacterial and fungal culture reports. The laboratory medical director may choose to add or delete information, depending on the individual case.

The infection control department may be able to help assess the situation, especially if the contamination problem is new or if the organism is a pathogen. This could include an inspection of the laboratory, focusing on an evaluation of procedures for sterile technique. Whether or not the organism is isolated from the environment, documentation of the investigation should include any procedural changes that are instituted. Consideration should be given to reagents or disposables as sources of contamination. The microbiology department can test aliquots of reagents. However, low levels of bacteria may not be detected by simply analyzing 5 mL of a reagent. The bacteria may have to be concentrated to allow detection. A large volume (500 mL) of the reagent can be processed through a sterile 0.22 micron filter to trap the bacteria. This filter can then be cultured to isolate and identify the organism. If software is suspected, one should place a volume of tissue culture medium in the disposable. One should remove the media, pour it through a filter and culture the filter. If a source of contamination is identified, both the manufacturer and the FDA must be notified. All conversations should be documented and the conversations followed up with letters.

Summary

Bacterial and fungal contamination of stem or progenitor cell collections is a concern because of the potential morbidity and mortality associated with the infusion of contaminated blood components. This is compounded by the fact that transplant patients are often immunosuppressed and may not have circulating granulocytes on the day of infusion. The techniques and reagents currently employed to collect bone marrow, peripheral blood, cord blood and fetal liver cells all are potential sources of contamination. Additional manipulation of these cells increases the risk of contamination. Reports show that bone marrow can be contaminated with bacteria during collection, processing and thawing procedures. Clinically, there has been only one reported septic reaction related to the infusion of contaminated bone marrow.

However, the incidence of contamination can be reduced through the use of good infection control and laboratory procedures such as hand washing, frequent changing of gloves and routine disinfection and drying of equipment (especially waterbaths). Efforts can also be made to reduce the risk of contamination by using cryopreservation storage bags with a low breakage rate and by designing processing systems with minimal cell transfer steps. The laboratory should begin to use a sterile connecting device in place of a coupler on open tubing connections to transfer cells from one bag to another. Finally, in the future, attempts should be made to use reagents that are approved for injection and to enlist the help of manufacturers to prepare and provide them.

References

1. Rowley SD, Davis JM, Dick J, et al. Bacterial contamination of bone marrow grafts intended for autologous and allogeneic bone marrow transplantation: Incidence and clinical significance. Transfusion 1988;28:109-12.
2. Thomas ED, Storb R. Technique for human marrow grafting. Blood 1970;36:507-15.
3. Lin A, Carr T, Herzig R, et al. Evaluation of a disposable bone marrow collection and filtration kit (abstract). Transfusion 1987;27:526.
4. Cameron S, Juni BA, Van Drunen N, et al. Reported contamination of heparin sodium with *Pseudomonas putida*. MMWR 1986;35:123-4.
5. Gilmore MJ, Prentice HG, Corringham RE, et al. A technique for the concentration of nucleated bone marrow cells for in vitro manipulation or cryopreservation using the IBM 2991 blood cell processor. Vox Sang 1983;45:294-302.
6. Van de Ouweland F, De Witte T, Geerdink P, Haanen C. Enrichment and cryopreservation of bone marrow progenitor cells for autologous reinfusion. Cryobiology 1982;19:292-8.
7. Yeager AM, Kaizer H, Santos GW, et al. Autologous bone marrow transplantation in patients with acute nonlymphocytic leukemia using ex vivo marrow treatment with 4-hydroperoxycyclophosphamide. N Engl J Med 1986;315:141-7.

8. Braine HG, Sensenbrenner LL, Wright SK, et al. Bone marrow transplantation with major ABO blood group incompatibility using erythrocyte depletion of marrow prior to infusion. Blood 1982;60:420-5.
9. Jansen J. Processing of bone marrow for allogeneic transplantation. In: Sacher RA, McCarthy LJ, Smit Sibinga CT, eds. Processing of bone marrow for transplantation. Arlington, VA: American Association of Blood Banks, 1990:19-39.
10. Noga SJ, Davis JM, Thoburn CJ, Donnenberg AD. Lymphocyte dose modification of the bone marrow allograft using elutriation. In: Gee AP, ed. Bone marrow processing and purging: A practical guide. Boca Raton: CRC Press, 1991:175-99.
11. Marciniak E, Bailey K, Henslee-Downey PJ, Thompson JS. Bone marrow purging of T lymphocytes with $T_{10}B_9$ monoclonal antibodies and complement. In: Areman E, Deeg HJ, Sacher RA, eds. Bone marrow and stem cell processing: A manual of current techniques. Philadelphia: F. A. Davis, 1992:208-10.
12. Rowley SD, Davis JM, Piantadosi S, et al. Density-gradient separation of autologous bone marrow grafts before ex vivo purging with 4-hydroperoxycyclophosphamide. Bone Marrow Transplant 1990;6:321-7.
13. Schepers KG, Davis JM, Rowley SD. Incidence of bacterial contamination of bone marrow grafts. In: Worthington-White D, Gee AP, Gross S, eds. Advances in bone marrow purging and processing. New York: Wiley-Liss, 1992:379-84.
14. Lazarus HM, Magalhaes-Silverman M, Fox RM, et al. Contamination during in vitro processing of bone marrow for transplantation: Clinical significance. Bone Marrow Transplant 1991;7:241-6.
15. Stroncek DF, Fautsch SK, Lasky LC, et al. Adverse reactions in patients transfused with cryopreserved marrow. Transfusion 1991;31:521-6.
16. Thorp D, Haylock DN, Canty A. Harvesting of recovery-phase peripheral blood stem cells using the CS3000 blood cell separator. In: Areman E, Deeg HJ, Sacher RA, eds. Bone marrow and stem cell processing: A manual of current techniques. Philadelphia: FA Davis, 1992:77-82.
17. Williams SF, Barker S, Hollingsworth K. Peripheral stem cell harvests in the steady and nonsteady states. In: Areman E,

Deeg HJ, Sacher RA, eds. Bone marrow and stem cell processing: A manual of current techniques. Philadelphia: FA Davis, 1992:83-6.

18. Cordle D, Koepke JA, Koontz FP. The sterility of platelet and granulocyte concentrates collected by discontinuous flow centrifugation. Transfusion 1980;20:105-7.

19. Rhame FS, Root RK, MacLowry JD, et al. *Salmonella* septicemia from platelet transfusions. Ann Intern Med 1973;78:633-41.

20. Book of Abstracts from the 2nd International Symposium on Peripheral Blood Stem Cell Autografts. Mulhouse, France 1991.

21. Gibson T, Norris W. Skin fragments removed by injection needles. Lancet 1958;2:983-5.

22. Kessinger A, Armitage JO, Smith DM, et al. High-dose therapy and autologous peripheral blood stem cell transplantation for patients with lymphoma. Blood 1989;74:1260-5.

23. Rhame FS, McCullough J. Follow-up on nosocomial *Pseudomonas cepacia* infection. MMWR 1979;28:409.

24. Broxmeyer HE, Douglas GW, Hangoc G, et al. Human umbilical cord blood as a potential source of transplantable hematopoietic stem/progenitor cells. Proc Natl Acad Sci USA 1989;86:3828-32.

25. Gluckman E, Broxmeyer HE, Auerbach A, et al. Hematopoietic reconstitution in a patient with Fanconi's anemia by means of umbilical cord blood from an HLA-identical sibling. N Engl J Med 1989;321:1174-8.

26. Wagner JE, Broxmeyer HE, Byrd RL, et al. Transplantation of umbilical cord blood after myeloablative therapy: Analysis of engraftment. Blood 1992;79:1874-81.

27. English D, Cooper S. Collection and processing of cord blood for preservation and hematopoietic transplantation. In: Areman E, Deeg HJ, Sacher RA, eds. Bone marrow and stem cell processing: A manual of current techniques. Philadelphia: FA Davis, 1992:383-5.

28. Touraine JL, Roncarolo MG, Royo C, Touraine F. Fetal tissue transplantation, bone marrow transplantation and prospective gene therapy in severe immunodeficiencies and enzyme deficiencies. Thymus 1987;10:75-87.

29. Touraine JL, Raudrant D, Royo C, et al. In utero transplantation of hemopoietic stem cells in humans. Transplant Proc 1991;23:1706-8.

30. Schafer TW, Everett J, Silver GH, Came PE. Biohazard: Virus-contaminated liquid nitrogen (letter). Science 1976; 191:24-6.
31. Rowley SD, Byrne DV. Low-temperature storage of bone marrow in nitrogen vapor-phase refrigerators: Decreased temperature gradients with an aluminum racking system. Transfusion 1992;32:750-4.
32. Stiff PJ, Koester AR, Weidner MK, et al. Autologous bone marrow transplantation using fractionated cells cryopreserved in dimethylsulfoxide and hydroxyethyl starch without controlled-rate freezing. Blood 1987;70:974-8.
33. Wingard JR, Merz WG, Saral R. Candida tropicalis: A major pathogen in immunocompromised patients. Ann Intern Med 1979;91:539-43.
34. Klein HG, ed. Standards for blood banks and transfusion services, 16th ed. Bethesda, MD: American Association of Blood Banks, 1994:49.
35. Perkins HA, ed. Standards of the National Marrow Donor Program, 9th ed. Minneapolis, MN: National Marrow Donor Program, 1993.
36. Blajchman MA, Ali AM. Bacteria in the blood supply: An overlooked issue in transfusion medicine. In: Nance SJ, ed. Blood safety: Current challenges. Bethesda, MD: American Association of Blood Banks, 1992:213-28.
37. Morrow JF, Braine HG, Kickler TS, et al. Septic reactions to platelet transfusions: A persistent problem. JAMA 1991; 266:555-8.
38. Walker RH, ed. Technical manual, 11th ed. Bethesda, MD: American Association of Blood Banks, 1990:471-89.
39. Davis JM, Rowley SD, Braine HG, et al. Clinical toxicity of cryopreserved bone marrow graft infusion. Blood 1990; 75:781-6.

/

In: Lasky L and Warkentin P, eds. *Marrow and Stem Cell
Processing for Transplantation*
Bethesda, MD: American Association of Blood Banks, 1995

4

Routine Methods for Preparing Hematopoietic Progenitor Cell Components

Charles S. Carter, BS; Ronald Gress, MD; and Harvey G. Klein, MD

BONE MARROW IS GENERALLY harvested by multiple needle aspirations from the posterior iliac crests and placed into a container to which has been added anticoagulant (heparin) in a solution such as Medium 199, normal saline or Hanks' balanced salt solution. Marrow is a mixture of peripheral blood (about 90% of the volume of marrow harvested by aspiration is plasma, red blood cells (RBCs), white blood cells (WBCs) and platelets),[1] committed hematopoietic progenitors, "stem" cells, fatty substances, blood clots and bone spicules. Marrow taken from patients with cancer for subsequent autologous use may also contain tumor cells. Marrow is typically harvested and filtered in the operating room and placed into a transfer pack for delivery to the cell processing laboratory or to the patient's bedside. The average volume of marrow is generally about 1 L, although the range of volumes is quite large (0.1 L to as much as 3 L).[2,3] Marrow volume depends on the size of the donor, the concentration of progenitor cells in the harvest and the number of cells needed for the recipient, which in turn depends on the weight of the recipient and the type of postharvest processing

Charles S. Carter, BS, Supervisor, Special Services Laboratory, Department of Transfusion Medicine, Warren Grant Magnuson Clinical Center, National Institutes of Health; Ronald Gress, MD, Head, Transplantation Therapy Section, Medicine Branch and Transplantation Immunology Section, Experimental Immunology Branch, National Cancer Institute, National Institutes of Health; and Harvey G. Klein, MD, Chief, Department of Transfusion Medicine, Warren Grant Magnuson Clinical Center, National Institutes of Health, Bethesda, Maryland that is planned. Marrow typically has a hematocrit of 0.20-0.25 (20-25%) and a WBC count of $10\text{-}50 \times 10^3/\mu L$. The quality of the marrow as measured by cellular concentration is critically dependent on harvesting technique.[1,4] Laboratories involved in the processing of marrow harvests must handle both large and small volumes, various amounts of packed RBCs, and from 1×10^8 to $>5 \times 10^{10}$ total nucleated cells.

Many factors contribute to the determination of processing requirements for each marrow component. Processing depends on donor type (autologous or allogeneic) and on recipient needs. Table 4-1 presents some of the reasons for processing marrow to prepare components customized for specific recipient needs.

Table 4-1. Determination of Marrow Processing Goals

Issue	Goal
Major ABO incompatibility	Reduce red cell content of marrow to prevent acute hemolytic transfusion reactions[5]
Minor ABO incompatibility	Remove plasma to prevent hemolysis of RBCs due to transfused antibody[5]
Small recipient	Reduce total marrow volume to prevent volume overload during transfusion
HLA mismatch	Reduce T-cell content to prevent graft-vs-host disease while protecting engraftment and graft vs tumor effects[6-8]
Cryopreservation	Reduce to a volume practical for freezing and infusion. Remove cellular elements that are often damaged by freeze/thaw such as RBCs and granulocytes
Fatty substances	Remove fat and other particulates that could cause an embolism or interfere with processing
Clotting or clumping of marrow during processing	Use additives such as anticoagulants (heparin, ACD-A, citrate) or enzymes (DNAase) or solutions (Medium 199, normal saline, Plasmalyte-A) to prevent cell losses due to clumping
Removal of contaminants that interfere with processes for positive or negative selection	An example would be 4-HC purge in which RBC contaminants interfere with the purging of tumor cells[9]

Each transplant center determines its own set of specifications for marrow components in terms of progenitor cell content, WBC content (nucleated cells, mononuclear cells, T cells, granulocytes), RBC volume and plasma volume. The goal of processing is the manufacture of a progenitor cell component that precisely and reliably meets these specifications. This chapter will focus on the more routine processing methodologies that remove bulk "contaminants" such as RBCs, granulocytes and plasma. After this type of processing, components are ready for transfusion, cryopreservation or additional modifications using chemical [4-hydroperoxycyclophosamide (4-HC) purge],[2,9-12] biologic (natural killer cells, antisense DNA) or physical techniques (negative or positive antibody-mediated selection or elutriation methods)[13,14] involved in cellular engineering of the graft.[15]

Early pluripotent progenitor cells are CD34+ cells[16] that segregate with the mononuclear fraction of WBCs and are the population of cells that need to be conserved during marrow processing. Investigators[17-21] have determined through isopycnic separation experiments that these cells reside in the light-density (1.060-1.077 sp gr) leukocyte fraction. Cell processing laboratories typically measure nucleated cells by automated electronic particle counting techniques or manual WBC counting. Nucleated cells may be further classified morphologically by microscopic examination. Most processing laboratories define nucleated cells as including nucleated RBCs, as well as mature and immature WBCs, although there is no standard definition. Progenitor cells are measured through their capacity to divide numerous times, producing colonies of 50 or more cells termed colony-forming units (CFUs) by biologic assays. More recently, mononuclear cell subset distributions, including CD34+ fractions have been quantified by flow cytometric analysis.

Methods available for routine cell processing may be categorized by three approaches: 1) differential pelleting, 2) rate zonal separations[17] and 3) isopycnic separations.[18,19] Differential pelleting separations utilize the differences in the size and density of the particles to achieve separation. Rate zonal separations take advantage of the differences in the sedimentation rates of particles. Isopycnic separations depend on differences in the buoyant densities of the particles.

Differential pelleting methods include centrifugation to remove plasma, buffy coat separation and inverted-spin techniques to remove fatty substances. Centrifugation to remove plasma and fat results in typical nucleated cell recoveries >95% of WBCs, RBCs and platelets. Buffy coat separation is a crude technique and results in a component that has many nonuseful cellular contaminants. Typically, the technique results in nucleated cell recoveries of >70%, and it reduces volume by 80-90% and RBC content by 85-90%.

Rate zonal separations include soft-spin (low g force) techniques for removing platelets with plasma and preferentially concentrating mononuclear cells in the buffy coat, sedimentation at $1 \times g$, which allows the component (progenitor)-rich plasma to be separated from RBCs, and techniques using apheresis devices, which result in the preferential concentration of mononuclear cells in the final component. Sedimentation techniques use agents such as dextran, hydroxyethyl starch or gelatin that increase the sedimentation rate of RBCs. These techniques result in nucleated cell recoveries of 70-90% and reduce the RBC content by about 95%. Techniques for enriching mononuclear cells by using apheresis devices yield components with 30-40% of the initial nucleated cell content and 55-80% of mononuclear cells, while removing >95% of the RBCs and granulocytes.

Isopycnic separations involve density-gradient sedimentation with reagents such as Ficoll-Hypaque, Ficoll-Metrizoate or Percoll (polyvinylpyrrolidone-coated colloidal silica)[18-23] to concentrate cells of a particular density. These techniques achieve the most thorough removal of RBCs and granulocytes. However, there is a significant obligate loss of committed progenitor cells, which may prolong the recipients time to engraftment.[24]

Numerous processing techniques and tools are available to cell processing laboratories, including manual and automated methods. Manual techniques involve "open" systems that use test tubes and working in biologic cabinets, or "semi-closed" methods that use standard blood bank technology developed for the collection and separation of whole blood using transfer packs. Automated methods use sophisticated equipment or devices, and are listed in Table 4-2. Ideally, laboratories should be proficient with both manual and automated techniques and thus should have the flexibility to work optimally with large or small volumes, different total nucleated cell content or varied RBC content.

Plasma and Fatty Substance Elimination

Use of allogeneic marrow may require the removal of ABO-incompatible plasma to prevent the infusion of isohemagglutins

Table 4-2. Automated Devices Used to Process Marrow

Device	Access	Type of Process	Type of Harvest	Extra-corporeal Volume (mL)	Minimum RBC Volume Needed for Buffy Coat Concentration (mL)	Isopycnic Separation Technique Published	Maximum Packed Cell Volume for Isopycnic Separation (mL)	Sterile Connection Using SCD-312® Device (Terumo or Haemonetics)	Comments
COBE 2991 Cell Washer	1 line	Discontinuous (cyclic)	Cyclic	75-600	50	Yes	200	Yes Large tubing	Requires a peristaltic pump for isopycnic separations
COBE Spectra	1 or 2 lines	Continuous	Continuous	227->1000	130	No	Not applicable	No Tubing incompatible	COBE 2997 cell separator not listed separately
Fenwal CS-3000	1 or 2 lines	Continuous	Cyclic	308 or 458	140	Yes	90	Yes	
Fresenius AS-104	1 or 2 lines	Continuous	Cyclic	120->1000	50	No	Not applicable	Not known	
Haemonetics Model 30 and Model 50	1 or 2 lines	Discontinuous (cyclic)	Cyclic	140->1000	120	Yes	150	Yes	
Terumo Stericell	1 or 2 lines	Discontinuous (cyclic)	Cyclic	140->1000	120	Yes	150	Yes	

that may cause RBC lysis. Centrifugation in test tubes using pipettes or in transfer bags using plasma extractors allows the removal of most of the plasma (about 75%).[5,25] Small volumes of incompatible plasma have been safely transfused into recipients of marrow and other blood components such as platelet concentrates. If more efficient removal of plasma is required to prevent a severe allergic reaction, the cells may be resuspended in an infusion-grade solution (such as normal saline), and this centrifugation step may be repeated to achieve >98% removal of plasma. When using transfer packs, the bags may be centrifuged with the ports upright as with a standard buffy coat preparation technique. The bag is placed into a plasma extractor, the plasma is forcibly transferred to another bag and the cells are resuspended.

To remove fatty substances, an inverted-spin technique has proven useful. Bags are centrifuged with the ports downward for the inverted spin. The packed cells are siphoned by gravity from the bottom of the unit into another bag, along with some plasma. The inverted-spin process allows the fatty substance in marrow to be removed most efficiently. Cell recoveries are usually >98% for both the upright and the inverted-spin methods. Fatty substances can cause problems with some of the automated devices by forming plugs in the tubing, which reduces yields substantially, particularly when using the Fenwal CS-3000 (Baxter Healthcare Corporation, Deerfield, IL) (CS Carter, unpublished observations) and the Fresenius AS-104 (Fresenius USA, Walnut Creek, CA) blood cell separators.[26,27]

Sedimentation Techniques at Low *g* Forces

Sedimentation methods add agents that alter the sedimentation rate of cellular elements of marrow. Wells[28] used dextran sedimentation for 15-30 minutes to reduce the volume and RBC content of marrow prior to a manual density-gradient separation to prepare components. Nucleated cell recovery after a single sedimentation process was 75%, and >90% of CFU-culture (CFU-C) were found in this fraction. Ma and Biggs[29] used dextran sedimentation in bags, siphoning the RBCs from the bag after a 30-minute wait and allowing a 2-cm thick layer of buffy coat to remain in the bag. Cells were resuspended and centrifuged to remove platelet-rich plasma. Recoveries were 71% for nucleated cells and 92% for CFU-C.

Dinsmore et al[30] reported a technique that used 6% hydroxyethyl starch at a ratio of 1:8 in 1-L transfer packs. Marrow was allowed to sediment for 90 or 180 minutes, and the component-rich plasma was transferred or expressed to another bag. Recoveries averaged 76% (range, 55-100%) for nucleated cells, and no differences were found related to time, although the top portion of the RBC layer was included when sedimentation proceeded for 180 minutes. RBC contamination was 17.8 mL for the 90-minute technique and 33 mL for the 180-minute method. Ho et al[31] reported a technique that added 6% starch at a 1:8 ratio and sedimented bags in an inverted position for 30-45 minutes at $1 \times g$. Red cells were siphoned from the bottom of the bag, leaving the plasma and a small buffy coat layer behind. Recoveries were 70% for nucleated cells and 55% for CFU-C, with residual RBC content ranging from 3.1 to 12 mL. Lasky et al[25] reported a mean yield of 90% for nucleated cells, recovering 60-100% of the initial CFU-C with a mean of 37.5 mL of RBCs using starch sedimentation. Warkentin et al[32] adjusted the hematocrit of marrow to 0.25 (25%) by adding tissue culture medium and then added starch at a 1:7 ratio. This mixture was allowed to sediment in the inverted position. RBCs were drained into another bag and were reprocessed by the addition of more tissue culture medium and starch. Their technique recovered 86% of the nucleated cells and 98% of the CFU-C. They were able to reduce RBC contamination to 0.4-21.8 mL.

Lopez[33] reported the experience in France with gelatin (Plasmagel, Laboratories Roger Bellon, Rhône-Poulenc Roror, Neuilly, France) sedimentation. Recoveries were 83% for nucleated cells, 82% for mononuclear cells and 80% for CFU-granulocyte/macrophage (CFU-GM).

Buffy Coat Preparation and Mononuclear Cell Enrichment

Buffy coat preparation takes advantage of differential pelleting by utilizing the differences in size, density and sedimentation velocities of RBCs, granulocytes, platelets and mononuclear cells. Progenitor cell populations have been found to reside in the mononuclear cell fraction. Centrifugation packs the cells tightly, and the component may achieve a hematocrit ≥ 0.70 ($\geq 70\%$). At this level, separation or layering tends to occur by displacement according to the density of the particles; erythrocytes and

granulocytes are at the greatest g forces (bottom) and mononuclear cells are at the lower g forces (top). This crude separation
concentrates ≥70% of the nucleated cells in the marrow into a
buffy coat and allows the removal of approximately 90% RBCs.
Plasma may also be eliminated during this process.

Buffy coats have been prepared manually in centrifuge tubes
or in transfer packs. After centrifugation, plasma is transferred to
an empty bag until the top layer of RBCs is within 2 cm of the
port. This portion or top layer of the RBCs (the buffy coat) is
diverted to another bag. This technique recovers 70-90% of total
nucleated cells while removing 90% of the red cells.[10,11]

There are many techniques for buffy coat preparation using
automated devices. Blacklock et al[22] and Gilmore et al[23,34] devised a method that uses the COBE 2991 (COBE Laboratories,
Lakewood, CO) cell washer. Harvested marrow was introduced
into the spinning container (donut or bowl) of the COBE 2991
device at 3000 rpm for 10 minutes; the hydraulic pump then
expressed plasma out at 100 mL/min and collection of the buffy
coat followed. Recoveries were 96% for nucleated cells and 91%
for CFU-GM with less than 25% of the RBCs remaining. This
component was processed further by density-gradient sedimentation prior to clinical use. Many other centers adapted modifications of this technique and report similar yields and recoveries.

Rosenfeld[35] adapted the COBE 2991 technique to reduce ABO-
incompatible RBC content by first collecting the buffy coat and
then adding 1 unit of washed, irradiated compatible RBCs and
collecting a second buffy coat. Recoveries were 77% for nucleated cells and 104% for CFU-GM. Incompatible RBCs were
reduced to less than 9 mL of the approximately 20-30 mL of RBCs
in the transfused component.

Mononuclear cells may also be concentrated by using the
automated apheresis devices listed in Table 4-2. These devices
use both sedimentation velocity and rate zonal separation[36]
effects to concentrate mononuclear cells, while removing >95%
of RBCs and >90% of the granulocytes. Methods are available
for the COBE Spectra, Fenwal CS-3000, Haemonetics Model
HV50 (Haemonetics Corporation, Braintree, MA), Fresenius AS-
104 and the Terumo Stericell (Terumo Medical Corporation,
Somerset, NJ).

Wiener and coworkers[37] developed a technique using the
Haemonetics Model 30 equipped with a 225-mL Latham bowl.
Marrow was introduced into the spinning bowl (4800 rpm) at

60-80 mL per minute. As the buffy coat approached within 1 cm of the bowl hub, cells were collected for 2-2.5 minutes. Marrow was processed twice in this manner. Recoveries were 63% for nucleated cells, 84% for CFU-C and only 12% for the final component. Braine et al[38] devised a technique with the Haemonetics Model 30 that used the 100-mL pediatric bowl. Marrow was introduced at 40 mL/minute and anticoagulated with ACD-A (8:1). When the buffy coat reached the shoulder at the top of the bowl, the flow rate was reduced to 20 mL/minute. Two 40-second or 13-mL fractions were collected. The final component contained only 5.6% (21 mL) of the initial RBCs with 55% of the nucleated cells, 75% of mononuclear cells and 57% of the CFU-GM. Linch[39] also used the Haemonetics Model 30 and pediatric bowl to process marrow. Marrow was initially processed at 100 mL/minute and then at 20 mL/minute when the buffy coat reached the bowl shoulder. The buffy coat was collected for 2 minutes. Yields were 75% for nucleated cells and 88% for CFU-GM.

Sniecinski et al[40] used the COBE Model 2997 to concentrate marrow. The apheresis kit was modified to eliminate the inlet and outlet filters. Extra ACD-A was added to the marrow to provide additional anticoagulation during the process. Marrow was pumped into the spinning belt (1100 rpm) at a flow rate of 60 mL/minute, and the concentrate was collected at 1.5 mL/minute. Mononuclear cell recovery was 88% and the final component contained only 5 mL of packed RBCs. Faradji and coworkers[41] modified the COBE Model 2997 to concentrate marrow using 900 rpm, an input flow rate of 50-60 mL/minute and a concentrate collection rate of 1.5-2.0 mL/minute. Recoveries were 26% for nucleated cells, 83% for mononuclear cells and 84% for CFU-GM. RBC volume was reduced by 98.5%. The COBE Spectra recently replaced the Model 2997 device, which is no longer manufactured. Davis et al[42] processed marrow through the Spectra three times at either 70 or 90 mL/minute with the collection set at 1.5 mL/minute in the manual mode of operation. The instrument's computer set the rpm according to the flow rate and the anticoagulant pump was set to 0. This technique recovered 22% of nucleated cells, 94% of mononuclear cells and 132% of CFU-GM. RBCs were reduced by 99%.

Areman et al[43] devised a technique using the Fenwal CS-3000 equipped with the Granulo separation chamber and A35 collection chamber. A computer program to harvest mononuclear cells was devised that was similar to the lymphocyte program, which used a pumpback step to clear the spillover condition. Spillover occurs when too many RBCs are harvested into the component. Before this report, two methods were used to correct this problem. The first technique slowed the plasma pump to a rate that allowed plasma to collect at the top of the Granulo chamber. The second reversed the pump, and 12 mL of plasma were pumped back to the Granulo chamber. Areman et al observed that, in the presence of tissue culture medium containing phenol red and nucleated red cells, the pumpback failed to efficiently collect mononuclear cells. The investigators modified the technique to pump only 2 mL of plasma back into the separation chamber and then stopped this pump until plasma had collected at the top of the chamber. The device was primed with saline supplemented with 1.25% human serum albumin and the filter unit was bypassed. Marrow was processed twice before the "reinfusion" step was initiated to collect cells once more from the separation chamber. Recoveries were 29% for nucleated cells, 53% for mononuclear cells and 76% for CFU-GM. RBC volume was reduced to 9 mL per component. Carter et al[44] used a modification of the lymphocyte protocol that slowed the plasma pump and set the interface detector to 75 to collect deeper into the RBC layer. Recoveries for this process were 65% for nucleated cells and 85% for mononuclear cells contaminated with a mean of 20 mL of RBCs.

Janssen et al[45] devised concentration techniques using the Terumo Stericell device. Marrow was introduced into the spinning bowl (4800 rpm) at 80-150 mL/minute. For the preparation of a buffy coat, when the cell layers reached the bowl shoulder the flow rate was reduced to 20 mL/minute and cells were collected when the effluent line turned pink. Alternatively, a surge technique or "elutriation" could be used to effect the separation of cells by switching the inlet from marrow to saline and then pumping saline through the bowl at high rates (>250 mL/minute) for the collection of cells. The authors found it necessary to use additional heparin to prevent clotting/clumping during the process. Recoveries were 53% for nucleated cells, 60% for mononuclear cells and 60% for CFU-GM. RBCs were reduced by 90%.

Zingsem et al[27,28] used the Fresenius AS-104 cell separation device to concentrate marrow. They used the P1-Y set and the Grancollect protocol, which involves cyclical collection of the buffy coat controlled by an optical interface monitor. Marrow was introduced into the spinning belt (1200 rpm) at 50 mL/minute, 400 mL of marrow was processed and a 12 mL buffy coat was collected during each cycle. Recoveries were 36% for nucleated cells, 47% for mononuclear cells and 68% for CFU-GM. RBCs were reduced by 93%. If results from patients with leukemia only (eliminating those with germ cell tumors) were analyzed, these numbers were 48%, 63% and 98%, respectively, for nucleated cells, mononuclear cells and CFU-GM.

Isopycnic Separation Techniques

Many of the components prepared by $1 \times g$ sedimentation or buffy coat/mononuclear cell concentration methods have residual levels of RBCs or granulocytes that may not be suitable for infusion or additional processing techniques. For instance, Rowley et al[12] found that the cytotoxicity of 4-HC was modulated by the RBC content of the component. As a direct result of this, they added isopycnic separation to the processing scheme to reduce the residual volume of RBCs as well as the variation between marrow products. Isopycnic separations generally result in the least amount of contamination of RBCs and granulocytes when compared to the techniques described above.

Wells used a manual technique,[28] diluting the harvested marrow 1:1 with Hanks' balanced salt solution and placing 40 mL of this mixture into 50-mL conical tubes. By use of a peristaltic pump, the mixture was underlaid with Ficoll-Hypaque (1.077 g/mL) and centrifuged at 1450 rpm for 30 minutes. Mononuclear cells were carefully collected from the interface using pipettes and washed twice to remove Ficoll-Hypaque. Ficoll-Hypaque causes RBC aggregation and thus increases sedimentation velocity; it is also hypertonic and causes cells to shrink because of osmotic pressure, thus increasing cell density. Wells' technique recovered an estimated 24% of the nucleated cells and 84% of CFU-C. Ekert et al[46] used Percoll to isolate a CFU-C-rich fraction of cells for transplant. Percoll is used at physiologic concentrations and does not cause cells to shrink or swell as a result of osmotic pressure during separation. Marrow was first concentrated into a buffy coat and then layered over 16 discontinuous Percoll gradients. Gradients consisted of 2 mL of 70%, 60%, 50% and 40% Percoll layered carefully one over another. Cells were centrifuged and the CFU-C-rich fraction at the interface between the 50% and 60% layers was collected and washed. Recovery was less than 20% of the initial buffy coat cells. De Witte et al[20] used a continuous Percoll technique to achieve a fraction (density of 1.0615 g/mL) that was enriched 25 times for CFU-C.

Gilmore et al[23,34] used the COBE 2991 cell washer and Ficoll-Metrizoate (1.077 g/mL) for separation of a mononuclear cell concentrate. Briefly, 150 mL of Ficoll-Metrizoate was placed into the container, and then marrow was pumped into the spinning device at 20 mL/minute. After separation occurred, the hydraulic press allowed the collection of cells at the interface. Recoveries were 25% for nucleated cells and 108% for CFU. Approximately 1% of the starting RBCs remained in this component. Lopez[33] reported similar results in France, with recoveries of 20% and 74% for nucleated cells and CFU-GM. Shinohara et al[47] reported a technique that used 200 mL of Ficoll-Hypaque with recoveries of 29% and 114% for mononuclear cells and CFU-C. Jin et al[2] used Ficoll-Diatrazoate with the COBE 2991 device and reported recoveries of 37%, 47% and 48% for nucleated cells, mononuclear cells and CFU-GM, with only 2.6 mL of residual RBC contamination. English et al[48] used 150 mL of Ficoll-Hypaque, but modified the collection by including the first few milliliters of the RBCs for the component. Recoveries were 37% and 58% for nucleated cells and mononuclear cells. Other investigators[3] have reported recoveries of 20-32% for nucleated cells by using slight variations in the technique for the COBE 2991 cell washer.

Humblet et al[49] introduced the buffy coat into the spinning Latham bowl (4800 rpm) of a Haemonetics Model 30 followed by Percoll (1.079 g/mL) at 5 mL/minute until the light-density fraction was forced from the bowl into a transfer pack. This fraction was washed in the pack once before cryopreservation. The final component contained less than 1% of the initial RBCs, 15.7% of the nucleated cells and 70% of the CFU-GM. Law and coworkers[50] used the Haemonetics Model V50 and Ficoll-Hypaque in a similar manner to isolate the mononuclear cell fraction. If a marrow did not have sufficient RBC volume to allow collection of a buffy coat first, it was subjected only to the density-gradient procedure (4/10 marrows). Law et al[50] recovered 28% of the nucleated cells.

Carter et al[44] described a density-gradient separation technique using the Fenwal CS-3000 cell separator. The buffy coat was initially concentrated into the A35 collection chamber. Then 40-100 mL of plasma was siphoned from the A35 chamber and the buffy coat was resuspended. Ficoll-Hypaque was pumped into the spinning A35 chamber and the light-density fraction was floated into a transfer pack. This fraction was washed using the A35 collection chamber before cryopreservation. Nucleated cell recovery was 28% and the component contained only 2 mL of RBCs.

Janssen et al[45] used the Terumo Stericell device for isopycnic separation of the mononuclear cell fraction of marrow. The buffy coat was mixed with normal saline and introduced into the spinning bowl followed by Ficoll-Hypaque (20 mL/minute). After 60 mL of Ficoll-Hypaque had been introduced, the pump stopped and the rotational speed of the bowl was increased to 5600 rpm. Ficoll-Hypaque was then pumped into the bowl until the light-density fraction had been collected into a transfer pack. The component was washed by using the same bowl. Nucleated cell recovery following buffy coat and density-gradient sedimentation was approximately 33% and contained 46% of the initial CFU-GM.

Summary

These techniques may be used alone or in combination to prepare hematopoietic progenitor cell components. As a rule, sedimentation or buffy coat techniques tend to contain more RBCs (10-35 mL) and granulocytes. Apheresis procedures with the Fenwal CS-3000, COBE Spectra and Fresenius AS-104 are able to substantially reduce granulocyte contamination through preparation of a mononuclear cell concentrate, although RBC contamination will remain approximately 4-15 mL. These techniques typically use reagents and supplies approved for human use by the Food and Drug Administration (FDA).[42,43] Isopycnic techniques will most likely be used only when there is the need to reduce RBC contamination to a minimum, usually 1-2 mL. Isopycnic techniques have the disadvantage of using reagents that have not been approved by the FDA for use in human therapy.

Automated processing methods for all the devices achieve remarkably similar results. Issues to consider before acquiring a new device include 1) cost of the instrument, 2) cost of disposable kits and reagents, 3) staff training (ie, presence of a staff member already trained for a particular device) and 4) availability of similar devices in the center (ie, the apheresis unit or blood bank) that could be used in the event of an instrument malfunction.

Cell processing has become an essential focus for preparing progenitor cell components for transplantation procedures. Research in adoptive immunotherapy and human cellular gene therapy will expand the demands on the cell processing laboratory. Many components such as gene-modified progenitor (CD34+) cells, antigen-specific (and functional) T cells or antigen-presenting cells may be prepared from a single product. Cell processing laboratories will need to concentrate various cell populations, place these cells into tissue culture for expansion and/or transduction and cryopreserve or store these components until needed. The challenge to these laboratories is to develop safe, efficient standardized methods that allow reliable definition of the biologic component prepared from each cellular harvest.[51]

References

1. Holdrinet RG, Egmond JV, Wessens JC, et al. A method for quantification of peripheral blood admixture in bone marrow aspirates. Exp Hematol 1980;8:103-7.
2. Jin N, Hill R, Segal G, et al. Preparation of red-blood-cell-depleted marrow for ABO-incompatible marrow transplantation by density-gradient separation using the IBM 2991 blood cell processor. Exp Hematol 1987;15:93-8.
3. Shpall EJ, Jones RB, Bast RC, et al. 4-Hydroperoxycyclophosphamide purging of breast cancer from the mononuclear cell fraction of bone marrow in patients receiving high-dose chemotherapy and autologous marrow support: A phase I trial. J Clin Oncol 1991;1:85-93.
4. Bacigalupo A, Tong J, Podesta M, et al. Bone marrow harvest for marrow transplantation: effect of multiple small (2 ml) or large (20 ml) aspirates. Bone Marrow Transplant 1992;9:467-70.
5. Petz LD. Immunohematologic problems unique to bone marrow transplantation. In: Garratty G, ed. Red cell antigens and antibodies. Arlington, VA: American Association Blood Banks, 1986:195-229.
6. Meyskens FL, Kiefer CA, Holmes DK, Gerner EW. Separation of normal human bone marrow cells by counterflow centrifugal elutriation. I. Morphological analysis and subfractionation of neutrophilic granulocytes. Exp Hematol 1979;7:401-10.

7. De Witte T, Raymakers R, Plas A, et al. Bone marrow repopulation capacity after transplantation of lymphocyte-depleted allogeneic bone marrow using counterflow centrifugation. Transplantation 1984;37:151-5.

8. Quinones RR, Gutierrez RH, Dinndorf PA, et al. Extended-cycle elutriation to adjust T-cell content in HLA-disparate bone marrow transplantation. Blood 1993;82:307-17.

9. Jones RJ. Purging with 4-hydroperoxycyclophosphamide. J Hematother 1992;1:343-8.

10. Kaizer H, Stuart RK, Brookmeyer R, et al. Autologous bone marrow transplantation in acute leukemia: A phase 1 study of in vitro treatment of marrow with 4-hydroperoxycyclophosphamide to purge tumor cells. Blood 1985;65:1504-10.

11. Yeager AM, Kaizer H, Santos GW, et al. Autologous bone marrow transplantation in patients with acute nonlymphocytic leukemia, using ex vivo marrow treatment with 4-hydroperoxycyclophosphamide. New Engl J Med 1986;315:141-7.

12. Rowley SD, Davis JM, Piantadosi S, et al. Density-gradient separation of autologous bone marrow grafts before ex vivo purging with 4-hydroperoxycyclophosphamide. Bone Marrow Transplant 1990;6:321-7.

13. Hardwick RA, Kulcinski D, Mansour V, et al. Design of large-scale separation systems for positive and negative immunomagnetic selection of cells using supraparamagnetic microspheres. J Hematother 1992;1:379-86.

14. Berenson R. Transplantation of hematopoietic stem cells. J Hematother 1993;2:347-9.

15. Noga SJ. Graft engineering: The evolution of hematopoietic transplantation. J Hematother 1992;1:3-17.

16. Civin CI, Gore SD. Antigenic analysis of hematopoiesis: A review. J Hematother 1993;2:137-44.

17. Miller RG, Phillips RA. Separation of cells by velocity sedimentation. J Cell Physiol 1969;73:191-201.

18. Boyum A. Separation of leukocytes from blood and bone marrow. Scand J Clin Lab Invest 1968;21:9-108.

19. Boyum A. Isolation of lymphocytes, granulocytes, and macrophages. Scand J Immunol 1976;5:9-15.

20. De Witte T, Scheltinga-Koekman E, Plas A, et al. Enrichment of myeloid clonogenic cells by isopycnic density equilibrium centrifugation in percoll gradients and counterflow centrifugation. Stem Cells 1982;2:308-20.

21. Kurnick JT, Ostberg L, Stegagno M, et al. A rapid method for the separation of functional lymphoid cell populations of human and animal origin on PVP-silica (Percoll) density gradients. Scand J Immunol 1979;10:563-73.

22. Blacklock HA, Gilmore MJML, Prentice HG, et al. ABO-incompatible bone marrow transplantation: Removal of red blood cells from donor marrow avoiding recipient antibody depletion. Lancet 1982;2:1061-4.

23. Gilmore ML, Prentice HG, Blacklock HA, et al. A technique for rapid isolation of bone marrow mononuclear cells using Ficoll-Metrizoate and the IBM 2991 cell processor. Br J Haematol 1982;50:619-26.

24. Kessinger A, Schmit-Pokorny K, Smith D, et al. Cryopreservation and infusion of autologous peripheral blood stem cells. Bone Marrow Transplant 1990;5(Suppl 2):25-7.

25. Lasky LC, Warkentin PI, Kersey JH, et al. Hemotherapy in patients undergoing blood group incompatible bone marrow transplantation. Transfusion 1983;23:277-85.

26. Zingsem J, Zeiler T, Zimmermann R, et al. Bone marrow processing with the Fresenius AS 104: Initial results. J Hemather 1992;1:273-8.

27. Zingsem J, Zeiler T, Zimmermann R, et al. Automated processing of human bone marrow grafts for transplantation. Vox Sang 1993;65:293-9.

28. Wells JR, Sullivan A, Cline MJ. A technique for the separation and cryopreservation of myeloid stem cells from human bone marrow. Cryobiology 1979;16:201-10.

29. Ma DD, Biggs JC. Comparison of two methods for concentrating stem cells for cryopreservation and transplantation. Transfusion 1982;22:217-19.

30. Dinsmore RE, Reich LM, Kapoor N, et al. ABH incompatible bone marrow transplantation: Removal of erythrocytes by starch sedimentation. Br J Haematol 1983;54:441-9.

31. Ho WG, Champlin RE, Feig SA, et al. Transplantation of ABH incompatible bone marrow: Gravity sedimentation of donor marrow. Br J Haematol 1984;57:155-62.

32. Warkentin PI, Hilden JM, Kersey JH, et al. Transplantation of major ABO-incompatible bone marrow depleted of red cells by hydroxethyl starch. Vox Sang 1985;48:89-104.

33. Lopez M, Andreu G, Beaujean F, et al. Human bone marrow processing in view of further in vitro treatment and cryopreservation. Blood Transfus Immunohaematol 1985;28:411-26.

34. Gilmore MJ, Prentice HG. Standardization of the processing of human bone marrow for allogeneic transplantation. Vox Sang 1986;51:202-6.
35. Rosenfeld CS, Tedrow H, Boegel F, et al. A double buffy coat method for red cell removal from ABO-incompatible marrow. Transfusion 1989;29:415-17.
36. Brown RI. The physics of continuous flow centrifugal cell separation. Artif Organs 1989;13:4-20.
37. Weiner RS, Richman CM, Yankee RA. Semicontinuous flow centrifugation for the pheresis of immunocompetent cells and stem cells. Blood 1977;49:391-417.
38. Braine HG, Sensenbrenner LL, Wright SK, et al. Bone marrow transplantation with major ABO blood group incompatibility using erythrocyte depletion of marrow prior to infusion. Blood 1982;60:420-5.
39. Linch DC, Knott LJ, Patterson KG, et al. Bone marrow processing and cryopreservation. J Clin Pathol 1982;35:186-90.
40. Sniecinski I, Henry S, Ritchey B, et al. Erythrocyte depletion of ABO-incompatible bone marrow. J Clin Apheresis 1985;2:231-4.
41. Faradji A, Andreu G, Pillier-Loriette C, et al. Separation of mononuclear bone marrow cells using the COBE 2997 blood cell separator. Vox Sang 1988;55:133-8.
42. Davis JM, Schepers KG, Eby LL, et al. Comparison of progenitor cell concentration techniques: Continuous flow separation versus density-gradient isolation. J Hematother 1993;2:315-20.
43. Areman EM, Cullis H, Spitzer T, et al. Automated processing of human bone marrow can result in a population of mononuclear cells capable of achieving engraftment following transplantation. Transfusion 1991;31:724-30.
44. Carter CS, Goetzmann HG, Yu M, et al. Semi-automated processing of autologous bone marrow for transplantation (abstract). Transfusion 1989;29(Suppl):6S.
45. Janssen WE, Lee C, Smilee R, et al. Use of the Terumo Stericell for the processing of bone marrow and peripheral blood stem cells. J Hematother 1992;1:349-59.
46. Ekert H, Ellis WM, Georgiou GM, et al. Marrow function reconstitution by fraction 3 of percoll-density-gradient separated cells. Transplantation 1986;42:58-60.
47. Shinohara K, Yamada K, Inoue M, et al. Improved method of separation of bone marrow stem cells by the IBM 2991 blood cell processor. Acta Haematol Jpn 1986;49:987-90.

48. English D, Lamberson R, Graves V, et al. Semiautomated processing of bone marrow grafts for transplantation. Transfusion 1989;29:12-16.
49. Humblet Y, Lefebvre P, Jacques JL, et al. Concentration of bone marrow progenitor cells by separation on a Percoll gradient using the Haemonetics model 30. Bone Marrow Transplant 1988;3:63-7.
50. Law P, Frantz S, Alsop T, et al. Processing of human bone marrow by an apheresis machine (abstract). J Clin Apheresis 1990;5:159.
51. Kessler DA, Siegel JP, Noguchi PD, et al. Regulation of somatic-cell therapy and gene therapy by the Food and Drug Administration. N Engl J Med 1993;329:1169-73.

In: Lasky L and Warkentin P, eds. *Marrow and Stem Cell
Processing for Transplantation*
Bethesda, MD: American Association of Blood Banks, 1995

5

Cryopreservation of Hematopoietic Stem Cells

Patrick J. Stiff, MD

T HE ABILITY TO DELIVER supralethal chemotherapy or chemoradiotherapy with an autologous bone marrow transplant (BMT) requires the ability to successfully harvest and store hematopoietic stem and progenitor cells. While hematopoietic stem cells can be kept for short periods at 4 C, the majority of transplants performed in the United States are done with stem cells that have been cryopreserved and stored at either –80 C in a mechanical freezer or at liquid nitrogen temperatures. While many advances have occurred in the selection of appropriate patients and the treatment of hematologic malignancies and solid tumors with autologous BMT, little has changed since the early cryopreservation studies of the 1950s and 1960s. These methods are effective, yet with the explosion of centers performing autologous BMT, care must be taken to ensure that methods developed in cryopreservation research facilities are quality controlled. This is particularly important, since there is still no Food and Drug Administration (FDA)-approved method for cell cryopreservation. This brief review discusses cryopreservation basics, and compares and contrasts the two major cryopreservation methods currently in use in the United States.

Cryopreservation Basics

The birth of cryopreservation occurred in 1949 with the discovery by Polge et al[1] that glycerol aided in the cryopreservation of

---

Patrick J. Stiff, MD, Associate Professor of Medicine, and Director, Bone Marrow Transplantation Program, Loyola University Medical Center, Maywood, Illinois fowl sperm. While glycerol is still the cryoprotectant used to store red cells,[2] for stem cells it was rapidly replaced by dimethyl sulfoxide (DMSO).[3-8] Recently, hydroxyethyl starch (HES) has been added to DMSO to help alleviate the damage caused by the freezing process.[9-10] These agents protect the cell from the lethal effects of the freezing process, primarily caused by intracellular ice crystal formation and high intracellular solute concentrations.[11-14]

For cells in suspension, cooling below the freezing point of water leads initially to extracellular freezing. However, "supercooling" or freezing point depression occurs because of solutes in solution (eg, sodium chloride) that depress the freezing point to approximately -10 C.[15] To -40 C, as freezing continues, intracellular ice crystals also form.[16] If the freezing rate is fast, these crystals grow rapidly, reaching a sufficient size to cause physical damage to cellular organelles and to penetrate the cell wall, causing cell death.[17] If, on the other hand, cooling occurs slowly to delay and reduce the size of these intracellular ice crystals, the resultant increase in the extracellular solute concentration causes cellular dehydration and ultimately cell death due to acid-base and biochemical changes.[18] In addition, physical damage to the cell wall occurs with slow freezing due to excessive cell wall shrinkage.

Cells that have more tolerance to the osmotic stress that occurs during freezing, such as lymphocytes and stem cells, survive this process much better than more fragile cells such as terminally differentiated granulocytes. While there is an ideal freezing rate for all cells, dictated by cell size and cell wall permeability,[15,19] it is clear that human cells, particularly hematopoietic stem cells, still will not survive the freezing process without a cryoprotective agent. With such an agent, intracellular contents become only mildly dehydrated, and the intracellular ice crystals are too small to cause cell wall and organelle damage. Small, permeable cells such as mature red cells are most viable when frozen at rapid rates, while hematopoietic stem cell viability appears optimal when cooling occurs at a constant rate of -1 C/minute.[20-22] Recent studies have suggested, however, that minor variations to this constant rate do not lead to substantial stem cell damage, as indicated by their clinical use.

In addition, cellular damage can occur as a result of the release of the "heat of fusion" that occurs during the phase change from liquid to solid. A lengthy delay during this phase change decreases hematopoietic stem cell survival, with the optimal duration being 1 minute.[23,24]

As frozen cells are warmed, the intracellular ice crystals formed during the freezing process actually increase in size, ie, they undergo recrystallization.[25] Their size is minimized by rapid rewarming, with optimal rates obtained by placing the cells in a 37-40 C waterbath.[16,20,22] This rapid rewarming also leads to a rapid dilution of the high intracellular solute concentration that is typically caused by the clinically used slow freezing rates.

Cryoprotective Agents

There are two main classes of cryoprotective agents, intracellular and extracellular. The intracellular agents used clinically are glycerol and DMSO, small molecular weight molecules that have the ability to diffuse across cell membranes. The extracellular agent used clinically is HES, which comes from a class of molecules with a high molecular weight, and thus acts on cell surfaces.

Intracellular Cryoprotectants

Intracellular cryoprotectants rapidly diffuse into the cell across the cell wall, thereby increasing intracellular osmolality during the freezing process, which minimizes the damage caused by both slow and rapid cooling rates.[26,27] For rapid cooling, the increased intracellular solute concentration leads to a decrease in the size of ice crystal formation. For slow cooling, rapid diffusion of intracellular cryoprotectants leads to a narrowing of the difference between the intracellular and extracellular solute concentrations, thus limiting the amount of dehydration injury.

Glycerol, still used for red cell cryopreservation,[2] was used for the initial studies of hematopoietic stem cell cryopreservation.[20,23,27-29] However, DMSO rapidly replaced it because of its ability to diffuse more rapidly into hematopoietic cells, and because, unlike glycerol, it could be infused to patients with the cells, thus minimizing postthaw manipulations.[3-8] The minimal concentration of DMSO necessary to cryopreserve stem cells has never been accurately established. However, the widely used 10% concentration, based on initial studies of RBC cryopreservation, is effective as measured by hematopoietic reconstitution after transplantation and is relatively nontoxic when infused into patients. Higher concentrations of DMSO do not appear to be more effective.[30] If in-vitro clonogenic assays are to be performed, the DMSO concentration must be reduced below 1%.[31]

Extracellular Cryoprotectants

These high-molecular-weight compounds do not have the capacity to diffuse across cell membranes. They appear to work by forming a tight barrier around the cell, decreasing the amount of intracellular dehydration seen with the slow freezing rates.[9,16,32,33] HES, the only agent in this group to be used clinically, has not been tested alone to preserve stem cells, but rather with DMSO to augment its capabilities.[9,10,34-38] As with DMSO, the optimal concentration of HES has not been determined. A 6% solution currently used with DMSO is the same concentration of this agent given clinically for volume expansion; thus, its clinical toxicity is minimal.

Combinations of Intracellular and Extracellular Cyroprotectants

While the initial study verifying the potential advantages of combining agents from the two classes of cryoprotectants was performed in 1968, it was not until 1983 that a potentially clinically useful combination was investigated. This combination, 6% HES and 5% DMSO, was initially used for successful cryopreservation of granulocytes,[39-41] which are characteristically not successfully preserved with DMSO alone. In marrow suspensions, granulocytes preserved in DMSO alone can clump, releasing nucleoproteins that in turn cause cellular clumps. These clumps may be the partial cause of some of the symptoms seen with marrow cell infusions.

Initial in-vitro studies showed that the total number and the viability of unfractionated marrow cells successfully cryopreserved in the 6% HES and 5% DMSO mixture were higher than the values for those in 10% DMSO alone, with a higher number of committed granulocyte-macrophage progenitor cells also preserved by the mixture.[9] No visible clumping was seen after thawing and intact granulocytes were easily identified on cytospin preparations.[9] For these reasons, this combination is being increasingly used. The combination also appears to be useful as part of a simplified cryopreservation process as described below.[9,10,34-38]

Both the traditional and simplified cryopreservation methods can also be used to cryopreserve peripheral blood stem cells without any changes in the cryoprotectant or method. Both methods do, however, require that a source of protein be added to the cryoprotectant mixture.[30,42] For cells cryopreserved in DMSO alone, this usually takes the form of autologous plasma at a concentration of approximately 20%. For the DMSO/HES method, human albumin is added at a final concentration of 8%. The added protein appears to act by stabilizing cell membranes after thawing, including the stem/progenitor cell membranes.[42]

Cryopreservation Techniques

For either of the two methods of stem cell cryopreservation in common use, the harvested marrow is initially centrifuged or sedimented with HES to deplete the majority of mature red cells. These cells are not successfully preserved by either method, and they lyse upon thawing. When infused, they have the potential to cause nephrotoxicity, especially when infused in large amounts or to patients with borderline renal function.

Cryopreservation Using 10% DMSO

Cells cryopreserved in 10% DMSO are done so using a standard method of rate-controlled freezing at -1 C per minute with storage in the liquid or vapor phase of liquid nitrogen.[6-8,31,35,43-45]

Many centers adjust the nucleated cell count prior to freezing to a final concentration of $30-40 \times 10^6$ cells/mL, because higher concentrations are associated with an increased incidence of cell clumping after thawing. However, at least one center now concentrates cells up to 8×10^8/mL and adds acid-citrate-dextrose (ACD) immediately after thawing, to minimize the formation of cellular clumps during the infusion of thawed cells.[46] After RBC depletion and cell concentration adjustment, the cells are cooled to 4 C, and the cryoprotectant (20% DMSO) is added to the cells slowly over a 10-minute period. The mixture is then placed in 100-mL aliquots in 300-mL polyolefin bags, and each bag is placed in a metal freezing frame, with a thickness of less than

5 mm. The frames are placed into a programmed, rate-controlled freezer, and cooled at 1 C/minute until they reach –80 to –100 C, at which point they are transferred to the vapor or liquid phase of liquid nitrogen. At standard cell concentrations, there are several aliquots of cryopreserved marrow per patient.

At the time of infusion, the marrow aliquots are rapidly thawed by placement into a 37 C waterbath and infused rapidly without a filter using an infusion time not longer than 10 minutes per bag to minimize the formation of clumping or gel formation. Washing the cells to remove the DMSO is unnecessary and may actually increase the chances of significant clumping, particularly if there are large numbers of granulocytes. DNAase can be added if visible clumping appears after thawing to dissolve the clumps.[47] ACD is effective in preventing clumps, but it will not dissolve them.

Cryopreservation Using 5% DMSO and 6% HES

Because of its ability to freeze granulocytes without clumping, this cryoprotectant mixture permits the cryopreservation of higher cell concentrations and in larger volumes. Marrow cells are concentrated as above, but rather than using a fixed concentration of cells, the volume is fixed at 300 mL. Cells can be successfully cryopreserved to at least 10^8/mL without clumping, although for the typical patient the cell concentration averages $30\text{-}50 \times 10^6$/mL. The cryoprotectant is prepared in advance by adding 42 g of intermediate-weight HES (mol wt of approximately 250,000) to 140 mL of Normosol R (Abbott, North Chicago, IL). [The starch is not available commercially but is available through the FDA through an IND for cryopreservation. Dupont Chemical Company (Wilmington, DE) is the current supplier of the drug.] The mixture is autoclaved for 20 minutes, which dissolves the starch and sterilizes the mixture. After cooling, 100 mL of 25% human albumin and 70 mL of 50% DMSO are added. For freezing, 300 mL of this mixture is added to an equal volume of cells in a 600 mL plastic blood bag. The cells are divided into 300-mL aliquots in polyolefin bags and frozen by simple horizontal placement in a –80 C freezer for freezing and storage as described below.

For infusion, the bags are thawed in a 37 C waterbath and each bag is infused, unfiltered over 30 minutes. Neither ACD or DNAase is added to the thawed sample prior to infusion.

Current Controversies in Stem Cell Cryopreservation

Do Hematopoietic Stem Cells Need To Be Cryopreserved in a Rate-Controlled Freezer?

The earliest successful studies of autologous BMT in animal models were done by immersing vials containing marrow cells cryopreserved in glycerol into glycerol-filled flasks, which themselves were placed into a dry ice bath. Successful reconstitution was obtained with these cells following lethal irradiation.[48] Subsequent studies using liquid nitrogen to control the rate of freezing explored the optimal rate at which to freeze marrow cells in glycerol or DMSO, as measured by nucleated cell recovery and colony-forming unit-spleen (CFU-S) assays.[20-23] The current clinical practice of freezing at –1 C/minute is a result of these studies, with the most important periods of the freezing process being the post phase change cooling rate and the duration of the phase change itself. While –1 C per minute was the optimal rate, increasing the post phase change cooling rate to 3 C/minute decreased the recovery of CFU-S by only 8%.[23] In addition, increasing the duration of the phase change from 1 minute to either 4 or even 16 minutes decreased CFU-S recovery only 16% and 28%, respectively.[23]

Recent studies exploring a non-rate-controlled freezing process were based on these studies as well as data demonstrating that granulocytes, platelets and lymphocytes could be successfully preserved by simple immersion into a –80 C freezer.[39-41,49,50] Minimal progenitor cell losses were expected, as this freezing technique produces an average 3 C/minute freezing rate.[9] In-vitro data using the DMSO/HES cryoprotectant supported this impression with essentially no loss of CFU-granulocyte/macrophage (CFU-GM) in the initial studies. Since most centers harvest and cryopreserve at least four times the number of nucleated cells as necessary to reconstitute hematopoiesis based on animal models, the minor amount of cell loss by this method as compared to 1 C/minute has been insufficient to detect a change in engraftment kinetics. Such has indeed been the case for the DMSO/HES cryopreservation method, with engraftment times similar to those obtained when cells were cryopreserved using the traditional method.[10,38] Successful non-rate-controlled freezing is not dependent on the cryoprotectant used, as clinical successes have been recently demonstrated for cells cryopreserved in 10% DMSO alone.[51] Thus, while there is an optimal freezing rate for hematopoietic stem cells, rate-controlled freezing is not required to achieve that rate and to preserve adequate numbers of stem and progenitor cells to lead to predictable engraftment following transplantation.

What Is the Optimal Storage Temperature for Hematopoietic Stem and Progenitor Cells?

As stated above, during rewarming from the frozen state, "recrystallization" (ie, the growth of intracellular ice crystals) occurs, which can lead to the death of the cell. To prevent this from occurring during storage, most centers hold marrow cells at the lowest possible temperature, which is either the vapor or liquid phase of liquid nitrogen.

Initial studies in a canine model demonstrated that bone marrow cells held at –80 C, or the temperature of a typical blood bank freezer, for short periods were just as effective in restoring hematopoiesis following lethal irradiation as were cells held in liquid nitrogen.[52,53] Again, cell dose appears to be critical, since storage at temperatures above that of the liquid state of liquid nitrogen is probably damaging, especially for cells held for prolonged periods.[52] In fact, as shown by Applebaum et al,[52] if the cell dose is at the lower limit of that required for restoration of hematopoiesis, even the vapor phase of liquid nitrogen was insufficient to protect against damage of cells held for 18 months.

The cryoprotectant used may be important in determining the optimal storage temperature. Since the damage described above is possibly due to rewarming, the use of the DMSO/HES combination with cells stored at only –80 C may be the explanation why both sufficient progenitor cells and pluripotent stem cells to permit reconstitution are preserved for periods of up to 2 years.[54]

Autotransplants after long-term storage are infrequent at any center, with most transplants performed within 2 weeks of bone marrow cryopreservation. However, the number of transplants done after long-term storage is likely to increase, with many centers now cryopreserving marrow in a "prophylactic" manner for patients with Hodgkin's disease and breast cancer. Caution must be taken when marrow is held for prolonged periods. At a minimum, small aliquots should be frozen along with cells for transplantation, and these aliquots should be thawed and assayed for progenitor cell viability prior to transfusion. Alternatively, a maximum period of storage could be established, with discard of marrow not used during this period.

For short periods of up to 6 months, storage temperatures even as warm as −80 C are sufficient to ensure prompt engraftment of cryopreserved cells at normal cell doses, ie, approximately 2 × 10^8 nucleated cells/kg. Beyond 2 years, care should be given to cells cryopreserved in DMSO alone and stored at temperatures above the liquid phase of liquid nitrogen. For the DMSO/HES combination, storage times up to 2 years at −80 C have been successfully tested, but the numbers are too small to recommend this without at least in-vitro assay of small aliquots to ensure progenitor cell viability.

Should Progenitor Cell Assays Be Routinely Performed on Cryopreserved Hematopoietic Stem and Progenitor Cell Collections?

Since the frequency of pluripotent stem cells in normal human marrow suspensions is less than $1/10^4$ cells, and since there is no rapid or simple assay currently available to measure their viability, most centers use assays of other cell populations to suggest that the pluripotent stem cell population is being successfully cryopreserved. Assays such as smears or cytopreps for histologic evaluation, dye exclusion studies, nucleated cell recovery and even committed progenitor cell assays have been evaluated, but in the vast majority of studies these tests do not predict for engraftment. Most centers currently rely only on a precryopreservation nucleated cell or CFU-GM dose to determine if sufficient cells have been collected and stored for a transplant procedure. This determination is based on minimum numbers of cells needed to reconstitute animals and nonhuman primates after lethal marrow injury. For all models tested, approximately 0.25 to 0.50 × 10^8 nucleated cells/kg are required.[4,52,53,55] Most centers have set a minimum of 1.5 to 2.0 × 10^8 nucleated cells/kg as the minimum number acceptable for transplantation, or approximately fourfold the number necessary. Based on the cloning efficiency of unseparated harvested marrow and on in-vivo data, this minimum cell number is the equivalent of approximately 1 × 10^4 CFU-GM/kg.[56] If these doses are harvested, patients who receive transplants should engraft with a neutrophil count >500/μL at approximately 20-25 days and platelets >20 × 10^9/L (>20,000/μL) at 22-28 days after transplant in the absence of posttransplant growth factor support.

While these prefreeze cell doses appear to be predictive of engraftment for the majority of patients, the postthaw recovery of nucleated and committed progenitor cells fails to correlate with hematopoietic recovery after transplantation. This is due to the fourfold excess of cells harvested and the fact that assays of committed progenitor cells do not measure the pluripotent stem cell pool. In fact, marrow purged with pharmacologic agents may be depleted of committed progenitor cells by up to 2 logs, but it may still contain sufficient pluripotent stem cell numbers to reconstitute hematopoiesis.[57,58]

Thus, the decision to proceed to transplantation depends primarily on pretransplant conditions: marrow cellularity, nucleated cell dose and committed progenitor cell assays. Nevertheless, some measure of postcryopreservation viability, while not predictive of engraftment, should be performed. Committed progenitor cell assays should be performed. If there is a consistent loss of >50% of CFU-GM after thawing of unpurged marrow, particularly if delayed engraftment is being seen clinically, the cryopreservation technique should be carefully reviewed.

Conclusion

The two current methods used to cryopreserve human stem and progenitor cells are equally effective in restoring hematopoiesis after autotransplantation. The use of DMSO combined with HES has permitted the development of a less expensive and more rapid method of cryopreservation in which a single technician can process and cryopreserve a marrow in approximately 1 hour. Long-term storage at temperatures higher than liquid nitrogen for this method remain to be more completely studied. It is imperative for centers holding marrow cryopreserved by either method for prolonged periods to measure the in-vitro viability before infusion. An overall quality assurance program is important for each laboratory that is freezing cells for transplant. More complete national guidelines should be developed and implemented as the explosion in new BMT centers, including those in smaller community hospitals, has meant that personnel without a research background in cryopreservation may now be involved in marrow processing and storage.

References

1. Polge C, Smith AU, Parkes AS. Revival of spermatozoa after vitrification and dehydration at low temperature. Nature 1949;164:666.
2. Smith AU. Prevention of hemolysis during freezing and thawing of red blood cells. Lancet 1950;2:910.
3. Ashwood-Smith MJ. Preservation of mouse bone marrow at −79 C with dimethyl sulfoxide. Nature 1961;190:1204-5.
4. Buckner CD, Storb R, Dillingham LA, Thomas ED. Low temperature preservation of monkey marrow in dimethyl sulfoxide. Cryobiology 1970;7:136-40.
5. Storb R, Epstein RB, LeBlond RF, et al. Transplantation of allogeneic canine bone marrow stored at −80 C in dimethyl sulfoxide. Blood 1969;33:918-23.
6. Wells JR, Sullivan A, Cline MJ. A technique for the separation and cryopreservation of myeloid stem cells from human bone marrow. Cryobiology 1979;16:201-15.
7. Weiner RS, Richman CM, Yankee RA. Dilution techniques for optimum recovery of cryopreserved bone marrow cells. Exp Hematol 1979;7:1-7.
8. Parker LM, Binder N, Celman R, et al. Prolonged cryopreservation of human bone marrow. Transplantation 1981;31:454-7.
9. Stiff PJ, Murgo AJ, Zaroulis CG, et al. Unfractionated marrow cell cryopreservation using dimethylsulfoxide and hydroxyethyl starch. Cryobiology 1983;21:17-21.
10. Stiff PJ, Koester AR, Weidner MK, et al. Autologous bone marrow transplantation using unfractionated cells cyropreserved in dimethylsulfoxide and hydroxyethyl starch without controlled-rate freezing. Blood 1987;70:974-8.
11. Mazur P. Cryobiology: The freezing of biological systems. Science 1970;168:939-49.
12. Pegg DE. Long term preservation of cells and tissues: a review. J Clin Pathol 1976;29:271-5.
13. Merryman HT. Freezing of living cells: Biophysical considerations. NCI Monogr 1961;7:7-15.
14. Merryman HT. Preservation of living cells. Fed Proc 1963;22:81-9.
15. Mazur P. The role of cell membranes in the freezing of yeast and other single cells. Ann NY Acad Sci 1965;124:658-76.
16. Leibo SP, Farrant J, Mazur P, et al. Effect of freezing on marrow stem cell suspensions: Interactions of cooling and

warming rates in the presence of PVP, sucrose or glycerol. Cryobiology 1970;6:315-21.

17. Mazur P. The role of intracellular freezing in the death of cells cooled at supraoptimal rates. Cryobiology 1977;14:251-72.

18. Bank H, Mazur P. Relation between ultrastructure and viability of frozen-thawed Chinese hamster tissue-culture cells. Exp Cell Res 1972;71:441-54.

19. Mazur P. Kinetics of water loss from cells at subzero temperatures and the likelihood of intracellular freezing. J Gen Physiokl 1962;47:347-69.

20. Bender MA, Phan TT, Smith LH. Preservation of viable bone marrow cells by freezing. J Appl Physiol 1960;15:520-4.

21. Leibo SP, Mazur P. The role of cooling rates in low-temperature preservation. Cryobiology 1971;8:447-52.

22. Mazur P. Theoretical and experimental effects of cooling and warming velocity on the survival of frozen and thawed cells. Cryobiology 1966;2:181-92.

23. Lewis JP, Passovoy M, Trobaugh FE. The effect of cooling regimens on the transplantation potential of marrow. Transfusion 1967;7:17-32.

24. Row AW. Biochemical aspect of cryoprotective agents in freezing and thawing. Cryobiology 1966;3:12-18.

25. Lovelock JE. The mechanism of the protective action of glycerol against haemolysis by freezing and thawing. Biochim Biophys Acta 1953;11:28.

26. Farrant J. Mechanism of cell damage during freezing and thawing and its prevention. Nature 1965;205:1284-7.

27. Merryman HT. Cryoprotective agents. Cryobiology 1971;8:173-83.

28. Pegg DE. Cytology of human bone marrow subjected to prolonged storage at –79 C. J Appl Physiol 1964;19:301-9.

29. Phan TT, Bender MA. Factors affecting survival of mouse bone marrow cells during freezing and thawing in glycerol. J Appl Physiol 1960;15:939-42.

30. Ragab AH, Gilkerson E, Myers M. Factors in the cryopreservation of bone marrow cells from children with acute lymphocytic leukemia. Cryobiology 1977;14:125-34.

31. Goldman JM, Th'ng KH, Pack DS, et al. Collection, cryopreservation and subsequent viability of hematopoietic stem cells intended for the treatment of chronic granulocytic

leukemia in blast-cell transition. Br J Haematol 1978;40:185-95.

32. Ashwood-Smith MJ, Warby C, Connor KW, Becker G. Low-temperature preservation of mammalian cells in tissue culture with polyvinylpyrrolidone (PVP), dextrans and hydroxyethyl starch (HES). Cryobiology 1972;9:441-9.

33. Takahashi T, Hirsh A, Erbe E, Williams RJ. Mechanisms of cryoprotection by extracellular polymeric solutes. Biophys J 1988;54:509-18.

34. van Putten LM. Quantitative aspects of the storage of bone marrow cells for transplantation. Eur J Cancer 1965;1:15-22.

35. Areman EM, Sacher RA, Deeg HJ. Processing and storage of human bone marrow: A survey of current practices in North America. Bone Marrow Transplant 1990;6:203-9.

36. Gulati SC, Shank B, Blank P, et al. Autologous bone marrow transplantation for patients with poor prognosis lymphoma. J Clin Oncol 1988;6:1303-13.

37. Makino S, Harada M. Akashi K, et al. A simplified method for cryopreservation of peripheral blood stem cells at −80 degrees C without rate-controlled freezing. Bone Marrow Transplant 1991;8:239-44.

38. Nademanee A, Schmidt GM, Sniecinski I, Forman SJ. Storage of unfractionated bone marrow (BM) without rate-controlled freezing is equivalent to standard technique for short-term storage (abstract). Blood 1991;78:251a.

39. Lionetti FJ, Hunt SM, Gore JM, Curby WA. Cryopreservation of human granulocytes. Cryobiology 1975;12:181-91.

40. Lionetti FJ, Hunt SM, Mattaliano RJ, Valeri CR. In vitro studies of cryopreserved baboon granulocytes. Transfusion 1978;18:685-92.

41. Lionetti FJ, Luscinskas FW, Hunt SM, et al. Factors affecting the stability of cryogenically preserved granulocytes. Cryobiology 1980;17:297-310.

42. Grilli G, Porcellili A, Lucarelli G. Role of serum on cryopreservation and subsequent viability of mouse bone marrow hematopoietic stem cells. Cryobiology 1980;17:516-20.

43. Appelbaum FR, Herzig GP, Ziegler JL, et al. Successful engraftment of cryopreserved autologous bone marrow in patients with malignant lymphoma. Blood 1978;52:85-95.

44. Spitzer G, Dicke KA, Litan J, et al. High-dose combination chemotherapy with autologous bone marrow transplantation in adult solid tumors. Cancer 1980;45:3075-85.

45. Gorin NC. Collection, manipulation and freezing of hematopoietic stem cells. Clin Hematol 1986;15:19-48.
46. Rowley SD. Hematopoietic stem cell cryopreservation: A review of current techniques. J Hematother 1992;1:233-50.
47. Salan SE, Niemeyer CM, Billet AL. Autologous bone marrow transplantation in acute lymphoblastic leukemia. J Clin Oncol 1989;7:1594-601.
48. Barnes DWH, Loutit JF. The radiation recovery factor. Preservation by the Polge-Smith-Parkes technique. J Natl Cancer Inst 1954;15:901-5.
49. Zaroulis CG, Liederman I. Successful freeze-preservation of human granulocytes. Cryobiology 1980;17:311-17.
50. Schiffer CA, Aisner J, Weirnik PH. Frozen autologous platelets for patients with leukemia. N Engl J Med 1978;299:7-12.
51. Clark J. Pati A, McCarthy D. Successful cryopreservation of human bone marrow does not require a controlled rate freezer. Bone Marrow Transplant 1991;7:121-5.
52. Appelbaum FR, Herzig GP, Graw RG, et al. Study of cell dose and storage time on engraftment of cryopreserved autologous bone marrow in a canine model. Transplantation 1978;26:245-8.
53. Gorin NC, Herzig G, Bull MI, Graw RG Jr. Long-term preservation of bone marrow and stem cell pool in dogs. Blood 1978;51:257-61.
54. Stiff PJ, Dvorak K, Schulz W. A simplified bone marrow cryopreservation method. Blood 1988;71:1102-3.
55. Gorin NC, Bull MI, Herzig GP, Graw RG. Long term preservation of bone marrow for autologous bone marrow transplantation (abstract). Clin Res 1975;23:338a.
56. Lewis JP, Trobaugh FE Jr. The assay of the transplantation potential of fresh and stored bone marrow by two in-vivo systems. Ann NY Acad Sci 1964;114:677-85.
57. Rowley SD, Zuehlsdorf M, Braine HG, et al. CFU-GM content of bone marrow graft correlates with time to hematologic reconstitution following autologous bone marrow transplantation with 4-hydroperoxycyclophosphamide purged bone marrow. Blood 1987;70:271-5.
58. Stiff PJ, Schultz WC, Bishop M, Marks L. Anti-CD33 monoclonal antibody and etoposide/cytosine arabinoside combinations for the ex vivo purification of bone marrow in acute non-lymphocytic leukemia. Blood 1991;77:352-62.

In: Lasky L and Warkentin P, eds. *Marrow and Stem Cell Processing for Transplantation* Bethesda, MD: American Association of Blood Banks, 1995

6

Malignant Cell Purging: Immunophysical Techniques

Adrian P. Gee, PhD

T HE SCARCITY OF RELATED HLA-matched donors for bone marrow transplants has prompted the use of autologous transplantation, in which marrow is collected from the patient while the disease is in clinical remission, stored frozen and reinfused following high-dose chemoradiotherapy. While this approach provides a potential source of marrow for many patients and avoids problems such as graft-vs-host disease (GVHD), there is a risk that the graft may contain occult viable tumor cells, which would be returned to the patient and may act as a source of disease relapse.

Although the marrow is usually harvested when the patient is in clinical remission, our ability to detect metastatic tumor cells within the harvest is limited. Conventional histologic detection methods have about a 1% limit of detection, which can be extended to 0.1-0.01% (ie, 1 tumor cell in 1000 to 10,000 normal marrow cells) by the use of tumor-directed monoclonal antibodies (MoAbs) and visual immunofluorescence or multidimensional flow cytometry. More recently, sensitivities of 1 cell in 200,000 have been described for immunocytochemical techniques, in which the specificity of MoAb binding is combined with morphologic examination of the stained cells.[1] Molecular techniques that exploit the amplification capabilities of the polymerase chain reaction (PCR) promise to extend this sensitivity

Adrian P. Gee, PhD, Professor of Medicine and Director for Applied Research, Division of Transplantation Medicine, Center for Cancer Treatment and Research, Richland Memorial Hospital, University of South Carolina, Columbia, South Carolina to 1 cell in 1,000,000 normal cells[2]; however, absolute quantitation of the level of tumor involvement remains a problem.

Assuming that an average marrow harvest contains 1×10^{10} nucleated cells, then, even when the most sensitive techniques are used for tumor detection, a "tumor-free" marrow may actually contain 10^4 to 10^5 cancer cells. There is no way of knowing whether such an inoculum would be sufficient to reestablish the disease, or in fact whether a single tumor cell in the graft would pose a significant risk to the patient. For this reason, several methods have been developed for the eradication of tumor cells from marrow that is to be used for autologous transplantation. This chapter discusses immunophysical methods for tumor elimination.

Tumor Purging Techniques

Many methods have been developed for the elimination of tumor cells in bone marrow grafts, ranging from hyperthermia and cytotoxic agents to immunotoxins and immunomagnetic separation.[3] All can, however, be classified on the basis of whether they physically remove the tumor cells from the marrow or destroy them in situ. A further subclassification on the basis of the use of tumor-directed MoAbs can also be applied. Immunophysical purging techniques fall into the physical removal, MoAb-based category.

Physical removal techniques have a number of advantages. First, by removing the cells, this method of purging avoids lysis of tumor cells and the release of lytic products into the marrow. In sufficient quantity, these products, such as DNA, can initiate cell clumping and gelling of normal marrow cells, making further manipulation extremely difficult. Second, immunophysical methods exploit the exquisite specificity of MoAbs both to identify the tumor cells within the bone marrow and to mediate their removal. These antibodies need not be tumor-specific, but may be directed to antigens that are present on the tumor cells but are not expressed by other cells found in the marrow. Antigen specificities range from neural cell adhesion molecules used in neuroblastoma purging[4] to high-molecular-weight mucins used as targets in breast cancer purging.[5] In every case the aim is to use antigens that are 1) universally expressed on all tumors of a particular histologic type, 2) present on the tumor stem cell and

3) not shared by the pluripotent hematopoietic stem cell population.

Disadvantages of immunophysical techniques relate primarily to the careful optimization required to ensure their efficient and reproducible performance. This includes the choice of component MoAbs in the antibody panel, the selection of their method of use, choice of incubation conditions and development of the hardware required to perform the physical separation of the cells. In most cases, tumor cell depletion is achieved by separation of the cancer cells from the graft (negative selection). More recently, with the identification of the CD34 antigen on primitive hematopoietic cells,[6] tumor depletion has been achieved by positive selection, that is selective enrichment and separation of the CD34+ stem cells from the marrow, leaving the tumor cells behind in the nonselected fraction. It is important to appreciate that for this approach to achieve levels of tumor removal comparable to those that can be obtained with active tumor purging, it would be necessary to enrich the CD34+ cells to >98% purity on a routine basis.[7] Few of the presently available stem cell enrichment techniques are capable of achieving this level of performance, with the result that tumor cells may be found in the stem cell preparation. Therefore, it may prove necessary to combine positive stem cell selection procedures with a negative tumor purging step, in order to minimize the risk of tumor reinfusion.

Physical Methods of Purging

Although purging by unit gravity sedimentation and elutriation do not strictly fall into the category of immunophysical techniques, they use some of the same principles and may be a useful adjunct to more widely used approaches.

Purging by Sedimentation

In certain cancers, tumor cells may have particular physical properties that differentiate them from normal marrow cells; for example, neuroblastoma cells are characteristically found as aggregates. These properties can then be exploited to separate the tumor cells, either by unit gravity sedimentation[8] (Fig 6-1), or by centrifugal elutriation (Fig 6-2).[9] In the former, the suspension

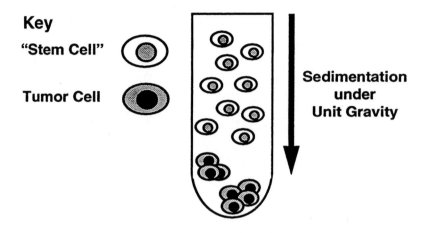

Figure 6-1. Separation of tumor cells by unit gravity sedimentation.

of nucleated marrow cells is left to sediment for a short period. Larger cells, including clumps of tumor cells, will settle to the bottom of the container, and the enriched normal cells in the supernatant fluid can be aspirated for further treatment. The efficacy of this method is highly dependent on a marked difference in the physical size and density of malignant and normal cells and at best will achieve insufficient levels of tumor depletion to allow it to be used as the sole purging modality. The efficiency of the method may be enhanced by further increasing the physical difference between normal and cancer cells. This can be achieved by using MoAbs to attach dense particles, such as plastic beads, to the tumor cells using tumor-directed MoAbs. Alternatively, floating beads can be used to pull the tumor cells to the surface of the suspension, where they can be collected and discarded.[10] Usually, these techniques achieve a maximum of 1-2 $\log_{10}$ of tumor depletion and therefore may be a useful "debulking" step to reduce tumor cell contamination to levels that can be addressed by more efficient and specific procedures.

Purging by Elutriation

Centrifugal elutriation is a sophisticated form of centrifugation in which cells are sorted according to size and density by balancing opposing forces of flow rate into an elutriation rotor

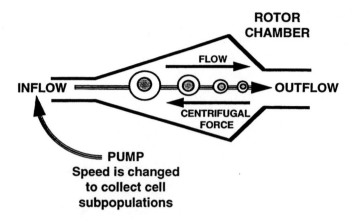

Figure 6-2. Physical separation of cells by centrifugal elutriation. This procedure requires physical differences in the size and/or density between tumor and normal cells for effective separation.

and the centrifugal force generated by that rotor.[9] The cells are then harvested from the rotor by adjusting either the flow rate or the speed of the rotor. This approach has been widely used to after the T lymphocyte content of bone marrow that is to be used for allogeneic transplantation. It has not found widespread application in tumor purging because of the variability in physical differences between malignant and normal cells. Although particles such as beads could again be used to increase the efficiency of the technique, this adds an additional level of complexity to a procedure that is already technically difficult.

Immunophysical Purging

Immunophysical techniques for tumor purging rely on the use of MoAbs both to identify the tumor cells in the marrow and to effect their removal. The antibodies may be added to the marrow cells in the fluid phase and the sensitized tumor cells collected onto a solid phase. Alternatively, the marrow can be directly incubated with a solid phase to which the tumor-directed antibodies have previously been coupled. Techniques differ primarily by the type of solid phase used and the geometry of the collection system.

Panning

Panning generally refers to a technique in which the MoAb is attached to a flat surface, usually a polystyrene sheet. The cell suspension containing the tumor cells is then incubated on this surface, during which time the cancer cells attach to the plastic via the MoAb. The normal cells can then be decanted or aspirated from the surface (Fig 6-3).

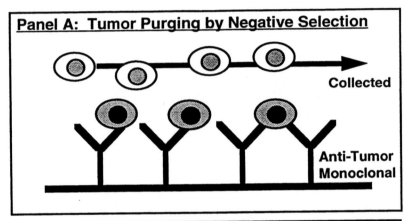

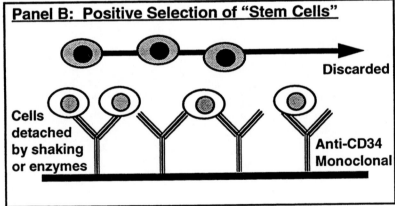

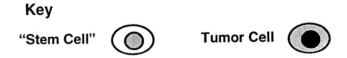

Figure 6-3. Separation of tumor cells (panel A) or hematopoietic stem cells (panel B) by panning.

Attachment of the MoAb to the plastic can be achieved by either passive adsorption or covalent linkage. The remaining uncoated surface can then be blocked by incubation with a solution containing protein, such as human serum albumin. The efficiency of coating by passive adsorption tends to be low, so that a large area of plastic surface must be offered to the cell suspension to ensure efficient capture of the target cells. Covalent attachment of the MoAb may substantially increase coating efficiency; however, the flat configuration of the surface still necessitates using a large area of material to achieve effective cell capture. This can become a significant disadvantage when a large marrow graft containing up to 10^{10} nucleated cells must be processed. As a result, applications for panning have tended toward positive selection of hematopoietic cells, rather than tumor purging.

If tumor depletion is the goal, then prior reduction of cell numbers in the graft by Ficoll-Hypaque density cushion centrifugation, treatment with soybean agglutinin or positive selection of CD34+ cells can effectively reduce the total cell numbers, making panning a more practical approach. Immunophysical separation methods offer the possibility of recovering the tumor cells from the solid phase for further study. In the case of panning, this may be achieved by physical disruption of the cells from the surface or by treatment of the attached cells with proteases such as trypsin or chymopapain.

Affinity Columns

The primary advantage of an affinity column purging technique over panning methods is the more efficient configuration of presentation of the immobilized antibody to the cell suspension. The solid phase in affinity columns usually takes the form of 200- to 400-μm diameter beads, and a 3-mL packed bed of these particles offers a similar surface area to that achievable with 600 cm^2 of plastic sheet. A variety of types of particles with differing surface chemistries may be used, allowing the antibody to be coupled either directly to the particle, or via a secondary immunoglobulin antibody using a range of chemistries. Alternatively, cells that have been treated with biotinylated MoAbs can be separated on avidin or streptavidin columns.[11]

Column separation methods tend (Fig 6-4) to suffer from the problem of nonspecific binding and trapping of nontarget cells.

This can reduce the yield of normal marrow cells and interfere with the efficiency of tumor cell separation. Interference with specific binding of the tumor to the solid phase may be reduced by exposing the cell suspension to uncoated solid matrix before passage over the antibody-coated particles. The cell yield can also be improved by extensively washing the column after the separation to flush out trapped normal cells; this will of course increase the final volume of the cell product.

Column techniques have not found widespread application for tumor purging, but have primarily been developed for the positive enrichment of hematopoietic cells. CellPro (Bothell, WA) has entered clinical trials with a system in which the marrow cells are reacted with a biotinylated CD34 MoAb and passed through

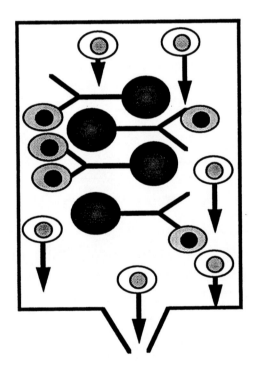

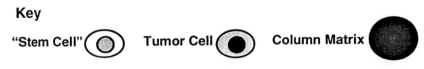

Figure 6-4. Separation by cell affinity chromatography.

a pre-column and then a column containing beads coated with avidin. The high avidity of biotin for avidin results in efficient capture of the CD34+ cells on the column.[11] These cells are then released from the solid phase by gentle stirring of the column bed. Adaptation of such a system for tumor cell depletion would require the use of multiple biotinylated tumor-directed antibodies to ensure maximal tumor cell capture, and the procedure would have to be optimized to ensure that immobilized tumor cells were not released from the column by physical disruption.

Immunomagnetic Separation

The immunophysical technique that has found widespread clinical application for tumor purging is immunomagnetic separation (Fig 6-5). In this procedure, the solid phase takes the form of paramagnetic microparticles that are added directly to the marrow, rather than being presented in the form of a column. The small size of the particles further reduces the volume of material that is required to offer the appropriate amount of antibody to the target cells. Depending on the size of the particles, anywhere from 0.3 to 1 mL of magnetic particles may represent a surface area equivalent to eight 75 cm^2 T flasks.[12] For clinical applications, two types of particles have been used: M450 microspheres (Dynal, Oslo, Norway) and magnetic microparticles (Advanced Magnetics, Cambridge, MA). These differ in appearance and properties. The larger size of the Dynal particles results in more rapid collection when they are placed in a magnetic field, but also in slower reaction kinetics with the target cells. The procedure used for cell separation is similar, however, for both types of particles. In contrast, magnetic microparticles and colloids behave very differently, in that they have an extremely high capacity to bind antibody, with the result that they can be added to antibody-sensitized bone marrow without the need to wash away unbound MoAb.[13] The primary difficulty associated with the use of magnetic colloids is that high-intensity magnetic field strengths are required for their collection. This necessitates the development of specialized equipment, which at present is not well suited to processing large numbers of cells. The biologic effects of free colloid that could be reinfused with the treated marrow remain to be determined.

In immunomagnetic separation of tumor cells from bone marrow, the normal practice is to add mixtures of tumor-directed MoAbs to a nucleated marrow cell preparation. This ensures maximal saturation of antigens on the tumor cells. Attempts to preemptorily attach the antibodies to the particles have generally not met with success, because of slower reaction kinetics, steric hindrance of binding of the immobilized antibody to the target antigen and difficulty in ensuring that the appropriate balance of antibody specificities is provided in immobilized form to each patient's tumor cells. Following sensitization, unbound antibody is removed by washing the cells, after which anti-immunoglobulin-coated magnetic particles are incubated with the cell suspension. The particles attach selectively to the tumor cells, which can then be separated from the marrow, together with any unbound particles, by passage of the cell suspension through a magnetic field.

Step 1: Antibody Sensitization

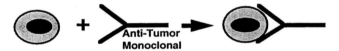

Step 2: Incubation with Magnetic Particles

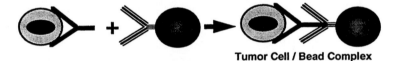

Step 3: Collection in Magnetic Field

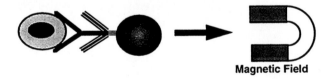

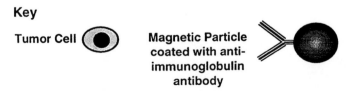

Figure 6-5. Immunomagnetic separation of tumor cells using the indirect procedure.

The disadvantages of this method are that it requires careful optimization in each application in which it is to be used, and studies have indicated that, while it is capable of separating cells that are resistant to other forms of purging (eg, complement) because of the low expression of the target antigen,[14] it can be adversely affected by binding very high amounts of the MoAb to the tumor cells.[15] The advantages are that a generic bead can be used to capture tumor cells that have been sensitized with a wide variety of MoAbs of different classes and subclasses, the system components are nontoxic to the normal marrow cells, and the small volume of the solid phase results in low nonspecific binding and trapping of normal marrow cells. This approach has been used to purge neuroblastoma, breast cancer and leukemia and lymphoma cells from bone marrow, either alone or in combination with cytotoxic drug purging.[3,5]

Preclinical Studies

The development of an optimized clinical purging procedure requires extensive preclinical experimentation.[16] A major factor in these studies is the selection of an appropriate model system that permits control of single variables during the process. A second consideration is the source of material required for these studies. It is usually not possible to obtain routinely the volumes of normal marrow that are required for an entire series of experiments. The most appropriate alternative is to perform the experiments in phases, in the first of which conditions are optimized for the small-scale separation of tissue-cultured human tumor cells in the absence of any other cell type. It is important to be critical in the choice of the tumor cell line(s) for these studies. Tissue-cultured cells may express homogeneous, high levels of particular target antigens, which makes them unrepresentative of the cells that would be found in an infiltrated marrow. Such lines may be useful in early experiments, in which antigen expression is not an important variable. Once the procedure is nearing clinical use, however, its performance should be validated by using a variety of lines, exhibiting a range of target antigen densities.

In the next experiments, the tumor cells are seeded into nucleated peripheral blood cells at known levels and the separation is performed. Under these conditions it is possible to label the tumor cells to assist in their detection after separation. Once satisfactory results have been obtained, the procedure is scaled up to process a clinically appropriate volume of material. Finally, human marrow may be substituted. This may be obtained as excess material from routine harvests, as cadaveric material or as material from bones removed during surgical procedures.[16]

Detection of tumor cells in the postpurge samples should utilize a number of techniques. Labeling of the tumor cells with a DNA fluorochrome that enhances their detection by visual fluorescence microscopy provides a sensitivity of 1 tumor cell in 20-30,000 normal cells. This may be extended to 1 in 100,000 by multidimensional flow cytometry.[17] Combinations of immunocytochemical staining and visual morphologic examination can result in sensitivities of about 1 in 200,000[16] and PCR can be used to provide positive or negative evaluation at sensitivities of 1 tumor cell in a 1 million normal marrow cells.[2] The clonogenic capacity of residual cells may be estimated in tumor colony assays, in which the identity of colony-forming cells can be confirmed by immunocytologic staining of plucked colonies.[16]

Clinical Procedure

The following is an outline of a generic procedure for immunomagnetic purging (IMP) of tumor cells.[18] It is provided as a guideline only, since it is important to optimize the conditions for each individual application of this technique.

Nucleated Cell Separation

IMP has been successfully performed on a variety of nucleated cell preparations, including buffy coats, enriched leukocyte fractions prepared by hetastarch sedimentation of erythrocytes and density-gradient-separated cells. Nonspecific cell losses during incubation with the microspheres average 20-50%, depending on the cellular composition of the cell suspension. Preparations containing phagocytic cells tend to show lower recoveries because the cells engulf magnetic beads and are sequestered in the magnetic field. This can be minimized by incubating the cells and beads at 4 C.

Antibody Sensitization

To achieve maximal tumor cell depletion, it is usual to use panels of MoAbs to detect and mediate removal of tumor cells from the marrow. This compensates for possible low expression of a particular antigen on a subpopulation of tumor cells. The selection of panel components depends upon careful screening of a large number of both primary and metastatic tumor samples for binding of the test MoAb in the absence of cross-reactivity with normal marrow cells. In addition, the selected antibodies should be screened for their effects on the functional activity of marrow colony-forming cells and long-term culture-initiating cells.

The concentration of each MoAb in the mixture must be determined in model experiments in which tissue-cultured or fresh tumor cells are seeded into marrow at predetermined levels of infiltration and sensitized with a range of concentrations of the test antibody, and the efficiency of depletion is quantitated. Because of the difficulty of accurately measuring the level of infiltration of tumor within a marrow harvest, the final antibody cocktail should contain a sufficient amount of each reagent to deplete approximately double the maximum anticipated tumor burden. As a general guideline, 1 mg of an active MoAb should be sufficient to deplete up to 5% of tumor from an average bone marrow harvest.

The nucleated marrow cells are incubated with the mixture of MoAbs on ice for 30-60 minutes with mixing every 5 minutes. The cell concentration during incubation should be standardized, and is normally in the range of 10^8 nucleated cells/mL, in either indicator-free tissue culture medium or normal saline containing a protein source such as autologous plasma or plasma protein fraction.

It is particularly important to wash away unbound antibody following incubation, since this will interfere with IMP efficiency by blocking the beads. Four washes with 250 mL of buffer are normally sufficient to remove fluid-phase MoAb; the final cell pellet should be resuspended to the desired volume to give the required cell concentration (normally ~5×10^7 nucleated cells/mL) upon addition of the bead suspension.

Preparation and Addition of Magnetic Particles

Prior to use, the magnetic particles should be washed extensively to remove any preservative. The buffer used for antibody sensitization of the cells may be used for this purpose, and the particles can be collected using a small permanent magnet. If paramagnetic microspheres are used, the concentration should be determined, by either an automated or manual hemacytometer count.

The optimal bead to target cell ratio should have been determined in preclinical studies. A general guideline is that 50-100 beads per tumor cell usually provides maximal tumor cell capture, and under normal circumstances this represents approximately one bead per nucleated cell. Therefore, the number of beads added should equal the number of nucleated cells being processed. In the case of other magnetic matrices, this calculation may have to be based upon volumes of the material rather than particle-to-cell ratios.

The appropriate volume of the magnetic matrix is added to the marrow cell suspension and the mixture is incubated at 4 C with slow (~4 rpm) end-over-end rotation for 30-60 minutes. Mixing can be accomplished using a rotating-wheel mixer adapted to hold a blood bag. After incubation, it may be advantageous to increase the volume of the cell mixture prior to collection of the beads. This reduces the bead or cell concentration and decreases nonspecific trapping of normal cells when the beads are drawn to the magnets.

Magnetic Separation

Separation of bead-coated tumor cells and free magnetic particles has been achieved using a variety of devices. In many cases, a combination of static and flow-through methods has been used. For example, the bag containing the cell suspension first is placed onto an array of magnets, which perform the primary separation, and the suspension is then drawn from the bag over another series of magnets that serve as a safety back-up to capture any escaped tumor cells or beads. The use of a disposable sterile fluid path is preferable to systems in which the separation chambers must be cleaned and resterilized. Large-scale devices have been described previously,[3] and commercial systems are available for research applications.[7] Again, the conditions used for separation must be carefully optimized with regard to separator design, flow rates, etc for each anticipated application.[7]

Assays During Immunomagnetic Purging

Before and after each procedure, the following assays are performed: total and differential nucleated cell counts; colony assays ± long-term culture-initiating cell assays; sterility; tumor detection (immunofluorescence, immunocytology, tumor colony assays, PCR, etc); hematocrit; and CD34+ cell quantitation. During the course of the procedure, total nucleated cell counts and sterility assays may be performed at appropriate stages.

Anticipated Purging Results

Under optimal conditions, IMP can achieve levels of tumor depletion that are at the limit of our ability to detect residual tumor cells in the marrow. In experimental systems, 4-5 $\log_{10}$ depletions of tumor have been reported.[5,16] Addition of other purging modalities may further extend the efficiency of purging. IMP has been found to deplete cells that are resistant to other forms of depletion (eg, complement),[14] and is unaffected by factors that can interfere with other purging modalities.

In model experiments, in which residual tumor cells were detected by blinded parallel fluorimetric techniques, immunocytochemistry and clonogenic assays, no clonogenic tumor cells could be detected in the final cell component, and there was excellent agreement between the detection methods.[16] In clinical experiments, this approach may also be used by combining immunofluorescent staining, immunocytochemistry and tumor colony assays. In addition, PCR-based assays are now available for a variety of tumor types. These are highly sensitive but are not yet capable of giving highly quantitative estimates of residual tumor within the sample.

Clinical Efficacy of Purging

From its inception there has been considerable controversy as to the clinical benefit that may be derived from purging tumor cells from the marrow. It is generally accepted that high-dose therapy is rarely, if ever, completely effective. It would be anticipated that after autologous transplantation, the majority of residual tumor cells would be associated with therapy failure rather than with infusion in the autologous graft. To date, a randomized trial comparing transplantation of purged and nonpurged marrow has not been undertaken for a variety of reasons. Many clinicians feel that such a study would be unethical if a method exists for removing tumor from the graft, and statistical analysis has indicated that it would be necessary to enter several hundred patients on each study arm to produce a statistically meaningful result. In the case of neuroblastoma, it has been estimated that such a study would take in excess of 20 years to complete. In diseases with a larger available patient population (eg, lymphoma and breast cancer) it may prove possible to address this question in randomized multicenter clinical trials.

Supportive evidence of the value of tumor purging has therefore been derived from a number of sources. Retrospective analysis from autologous transplants for acute myelogenous leukemia in Europe indicated that patients receiving purged marrow did significantly better, although the patient group was extremely heterogeneous.[19] More recently, improved survival was reported in lymphoma patients who received marrow that was purged to PCR-negativity as compared to patients whose grafts still contained tumor as detected with this assay.[20] Another approach being used to address this question is that of gene marking. A number of investigators are using retroviral vectors to introduce marker genes into tumor cells in autologous marrow grafts with the aim of determining whether marked cells can be detected at the site of disease relapse following transplantation.

In acute myelogenous leukemia and neuroblastoma, Brenner et al[21] were able to find tumor cells marked with a neomycin-resistance gene in patients whose disease has relapsed, which suggests that these infused cells in the graft may be associated with recurrence, although it may be argued that the marked cells have homed to a particularly favorable site (see Chapter 8). In a parallel protocol, the aim will be to mark aliquots of marrow with two different neomycin-resistance genes. One aliquot will then be purged, remixed with the unpurged sample and transplanted to the patient. At the time of relapse, the tumor cells will be examined for the presence of the two markers. If no markers are detected then no conclusions may be drawn. If only the marker used to tag cells in the unpurged aliquot is detected, this suggests that infused tumor cells may be associated with disease relapse and that tumor cells in the purged aliquot were removed by the purging procedure. If both markers are detected at the time of recurrence this indicates that the purging procedure has been ineffective and requires improvement.

Future Studies

Immunophysical techniques have provided a core technology for tumor cell purging; however, considerable controversy remains regarding the clinical value of this procedure. Ongoing studies using gene marking and planned clinical trials may eventually provide a definitive answer. In the interim, the practice has been for many centers to include a purging procedure, provided that it does not pose a significant additional risk to the patients. In the United States, this has been of some concern to the Food and Drug Administration, which has been anxious to determine whether this procedure confers any clinical benefit.

One approach to circumventing the issue was to emphasize the use of enriched stem cells for autologous transplantation. It was reasoned that purification of CD34+ cells would result in a concomitant decrease in tumor cell contamination of the graft, that would obviate the need for tumor purging. In practice, it may be necessary to achieve greater than 98% pure CD34+ cells to achieve a level of tumor depletion comparable to that obtainable with an active tumor purging procedure.[7] Most current stem cell enrichment methods are not capable of achieving this level of purity on a routine basis, and preliminary results have indicated that the "stem cell" preparations that are now being used may contain tumor. This suggests that it may be necessary to combine a positive stem cell enrichment procedure with a negative tumor depletion step. In this case, the tumor depletion step would now be perfomed on small scale using the CD34-selected population as the starting material. Potentially, this would make the procedure both simpler and faster.

One complication that must be addressed, if immunomagnetic separation is used to provide the CD34-enriched cells, is that chymopapain is presently used to detach the "stem cells" from the paramagnetic beads. This enzyme digests an epitope on the CD34 antigen, thereby releasing the cell. However, it also attacks other antigens on the surface of cells, including some tumor-associated markers that would be useful for purging any residual cancer cells from the CD34+ population. To overcome this problem, it would be necessary either to perform the purging step first or to use a different procedure to prepare the stem cell suspension.

A second major area of interest is the use of peripheral blood stem cells to replace bone marrow for autologous transplantation. The use of cyclophosphamide in combination with recombinant human growth factors allows CD34+ cells to be mobilized into the peripheral blood, from which they may be harvested by leukapheresis. This approach may also obviate the necessity to purge, since the incidence of tumor cells in the peripheral blood is expected to be markedly less than that in the marrow. A number of ongoing studies are directed toward determining whether this is indeed the case.[22] In a study of 48 patients with breast cancer, tumor involvement of the marrow was seen in 66.7% of cases and in 9.8% of cases breast cancer cells were also detected in the peripheral blood (Ross AA, personal communication), and in each case the level of infiltration was markedly lower. Additional data will be needed to confirm these findings; however, these results raise the questions of what number of tumor cells can be safely returned to a patent, and should we consider purging peripheral blood stem cell preparations? An alternative approach may be to perform a CD34-enrichment procedure, which would both reduce the considerable volume of the peripheral blood stem cell material and may serve to provide a useful level of tumor reduction.

In conclusion, immunophysical cell separation techniques have found widespread application for the depletion of tumor cells from autologous bone marrow, and many techniques have now been adapted for the enrichment of CD34+ cells for "stem cell" transplants. A number of issues remain to be resolved, including the sensitive detection of residual tumor cells, the clinical value of purging and the question of whether "stem cell"-enriched preparations from either bone marrow or blood should be purged of tumor cells. These methods for graft engineering have developed rapidly, and the resolution of some of these questions should ensure a strong and varied future for this approach.

References

1. Moss TJ, Reynolds CP, Sather HN, et al. Prognostic value of immunocytologic detection of bone marrow metastases in neuroblastoma. N Engl J Med 1991;324:219-26.
2. Mattano LA, Moss TJ, Emerson SG. Sensitive detection of rare circulating neuroblastoma cells by the reverse transcriptase-polymerase chain reaction. Cancer Res 1992;52:4701-5.

3. Worthington-White D, Gee AP, Gross S, eds. Advances in bone marrow purging and processing. New York: Wiley-Liss, 1991.
4. Kemshead JT. Immunomagnetic manipulation of hematopoietic cells. J Hematother 1992;1:35-44.
5. Shpall EJ, Bast RC, Johnston CS, et al. Combined purging approaches in autologous transplantation. In: Gee AP, ed. Bone marrow processing and purging. Boca Raton, FL: CRC Press, 1991:307-28.
6. Civin CI, Strauss LC, Brovall C, et al. Antigenic analysis of hematopoiesis III. A hematopoietic progenitor cell surface antigen defined by a monoclonal antibody raised against KG-1a cells. J Immunol 1984;133:157-65.
7. Hardwick RA, Kulcinski D, Mansour V, et al. Design of large-scale separation systems for positive and negative immunomagnetic selection of cells using supermagnetic microspheres. J Hematother 1992;1:379-86.
8. Reynolds CP, Seeger RC, Vo JJ, et al. Purging of bone marrow with immunomagnetic beads: Studies with neuroblastoma as a model system. In: Dicke KA, Spitzer G, Zander AR, eds. Autologous bone marrow transplantation. Houston, TX: The University of Texas M. D. Anderson Hospital and Tumor Institute at Houston, 1985:439-47.
9. Noga S, Davis J, Thoburn C, Donnenberg A. Lymphocyte dose modification of the bone marrow using elutriation. In: Gee AP, ed. Bone marrow processing and purging. Boca Raton, FL: CRC Press, 1991:175-200.
10. Hirn-Scavennec J, Brailly H, Maraninchi D, et al. Elimination of leukemic cells from human bone marrow using floating beads. Transplantation 1988;46:558-63.
11. Berenson R. Transplantation of hematopoietic stem cells. J Hematother 1993;2:347-9.
12. Lansdorp PM, Thomas TE, Schmidt CR, Eaves CJ. Marrow contamination: Positive selection. In: Armitage JO, Antman KH, eds. High-dose cancer therapy. Baltimore, MD: Williams and Wilkins, 1992:276-88.
13. Liberti PA, Feeley BP. Ferrofluid as a matrix for magnetic separations. In: Kemshead JT, ed. Magnetic separation techniques applied to cellular and molecular biology. Somerset, UK: Wordsmith's Conference Publications, 1991:47-54.
14. Janssen WE, Lee C, Gross S, Gee AP. Low antigen density leukemia cells: Selection and comparative resistance to an-

tibody-mediated marrow purging. Exp Hematol 1989;17:252-7.

15. Gee AP, Mansour VH, Weiler MB. Effects of target antigen density on the efficacy of immunomagnetic cell separation. J Immunol Methods 1991;142:127-33.

16. Gee AP, Moss TJ, Mansour VH, et al. Large scale immunomagnetic separation system for the removal of tumor cells from bone marrow. In: Worthington-White D, Gee AP, Gross S, eds. Advances in bone marrow purging and processing. New York: Wiley-Liss, 1991:181-7.

17. Stelzer GT, Shults KE, Wormsley SB, Loken MR. Detection of occult lymphoma cells in bone marrow aspirates by multi-dimensional flow cytometry. In: Worthington-White D, Gee AP, Gross S, eds. Advances in bone marrow purging and processing. New York: Wiley-Liss, 1991:629-35.

18. Gee AP, Gross S, Graham-Pole J, Lee C. Immunomagnetic purging of neuroblastoma cells from autologous bone marrow. In: Areman E, Deeg HJ, Sacher RA, eds. Bone marrow and stem cell processing: A manual of current techniques. Philadelphia: F. A. Davis, 1992:267-74.

19. Gorin NC, Aegerter P, Auvert B, et al. Autologous bone marrow transplantation for acute myelocytic leukemia in first remission: A European survey of the role of marrow purging. Blood 1990;75:1606-14.

20. Gribben JG, Freedman AS, Neuberg D, et al. Immunologic purging of marrow assessed by PCR before autologus bone marrow transplantation for B cell lymphoma. N Engl J Med 1992;325:1525-33.

21. Brenner MK, Rill DR, Moen RC, et al. Gene-marking to trace origin of relapse after autologous bone-marrow transplantation. Lancet 1993;341:85-6.

22. Moss TJ, Ross AA. The risk of tumor cell contamination in peripheral blood stem cell collections. J Hematother 1992;1:225-32.

In: Lasky L and Warkentin P, eds. *Marrow and Stem Cell
Processing for Transplantation*
Bethesda, MD: American Association of Blood Banks, 1995

7

Malignant Cell Purging: Monoclonal Antibodies

Kenneth C. Anderson, MD

MONOCLONAL ANTIBODIES (MoAbs) that bind to antigens on the surface of malignant cells have been characterized. These antibodies have been a useful complement to histopathology for the diagnosis and classification of
malignancies of both hematologic and solid tumor origin.[1] They
have permitted identification of the normal cellular counterpart
of malignancies, eg, the correlation of non-T-cell acute lymphocytic leukemia as a tumor of pre-B cells,[2] and permitted isolation
and purification of tumor cells for in-vitro study of their functional repertoire and growth regulation.[3] They have been employed systemically to target tumor cells in-vivo (serotherapy)[4]
and utilized in vitro to deplete antigen-bearing cells from marrow,[5]
eg, T cells from allografts or tumor cells from autografts. Their
precise role in the therapy of malignancies remains to be defined.

In-Vivo Use of Monoclonal Antibodies

In-vivo serotherapy has been attempted with MoAbs alone;
MoAbs conjugated to toxins, ie, immunotoxins; and MoAbs
bound to radionuclides. There are several obstacles to serotherapy regardless of the agent employed. First, one may not
be able to deliver the MoAb to the tumor because of tumor bulk,
nonspecific MoAb binding to normal tissues, antigen shedding

Kenneth C. Anderson, MD, Medical Director, Blood Component Laboratory,
Dana-Farber Cancer Institute and Associate Professor of Medicine, Harvard
Medical School, Boston, Massachusetts
(Supported by National Institutes of Health, Grant CA50947.)

or antigen modulation. Since no antigens are uniquely expressed on malignant cells, rigorous histopathologic screening for reactivity of MoAbs on various normal human tissues and toxicity trials using animal models are required, whenever possible, prior to their use in humans. If the target antigen is shed or internalized from the cell surface, MoAb targeting will obviously be ineffective.

A second potential problem with serotherapy is the binding of MoAb to tumor cells, but with ineffective killing. MoAbs may bind to antigens and activate either complement cytotoxicity or antibody-dependent cellular cytotoxicity. In addition, the binding of MoAbs to antigen on the tumor cell surface may result in Fc-mediated binding of macrophages and release of cytokines, ie, tumor necrosis factor or interleukin-1, from these bound cells. MoAbs bound to antigens on the tumor cell surface may exert direct effects, eg, MoAb directed against a growth factor receptor may have direct antiproliferative effects. MoAbs against a growth factor may be useful; eg, anti-interleukin-6 MoAb can transiently clear tumor cells and related clinical manifestations in patients with multiple myeloma.[6] Since there is heterogeneity of cell surface antigen expression within a given malignancy,[7] the MoAb utilized may not target all tumor cells and, in particular, may not react with clonogenic tumor cells. Finally, given the heterogeneity of cell surface phenotype within a given patient, there may be emergence of antigen-negative tumor cells, which would escape serotherapy.

A third potential disadvantage of serotherapy is related to its toxicities. Since MoAbs are usually produced in mice, their administration to humans may be complicated by reactions in patients with allergies to mouse proteins. Moreover, their repeated administration may lead to the formation of antibodies to mouse immunoglobulin, precluding their further use. More important, nonspecific binding of MoAb can lead to immediate and long-term end-organ damage. Indeed, adverse reactions to infusions of murine MoAbs have been observed in one third of patients. Fevers, rigors and diaphoresis have been reported in 20%; hypersensitivity reactions with urticaria, pruritus and bronchospasm in 18%; and anaphylaxis only rarely.[8]

To date, the results of clinical trials using unconjugated MoAbs as serotherapy for patients with malignancies have been disappointing, with responses usually incomplete and transient. There are a few promising reports. Brown and colleagues[9] observed a complete remission lasting several years and other responses of short duration in recipients of anti-idiotypic antibodies to their B-cell malignancies. Another promising report is that of Waldman and coworkers,[10] who described three complete and three partial responses in patients with adult T-cell leukemia-lymphoma who received MoAb directed against the interleukin-2 receptor. Nonetheless, the above described problems with MoAb delivery, phenotypic heterogeneity of tumor cells and toxicity remain inherent to this approach.

To enhance the cytotoxicity of unconjugated MoAbs, these reagents have been conjugated to either toxins or nuclides. Antibody-toxin conjugates can be formed by using highly potent protein toxins that can kill 5 $\log_{10}$ of antigen-bearing cells.[4] Because of their high potency, small (nanomolar) concentrations may be effective. Obviously, the target antigen must be solely or preferentially expressed on malignant cells. In addition, the antigen ideally should be internalized after MoAb binding to facilitate transfer of the toxin to the cytoplasm of the cell. To date the major toxins utilized are ricin,[11,12] diphtheria toxin[13,14] and pseudomonas exotoxin. [15,16] Although all are potent inhibitors of protein synthesis, they have different mechanisms of action. The A chain of ricin acts catalytically on the 60S ribosomal subunit, whereas the B chain mediates nonspecific binding of toxin to the cell and assists in the translocation of the A chain into the cytoplasm. The A chain of diphtheria toxin inactivates elongation factor 2, and the B chain mediates both nonspecific binding to cells and toxin translocation. Pseudomonas exotoxin has domains I, II and III, which mediate binding, toxin translocation and elongation factor 2 inactivation, respectively. In each case, the nonspecific binding can be decreased by alterations in the binding domain.

In clinical trials of immunotoxins to date, the most common toxicity is capillary leak syndrome, characterized by weight gain, peripheral edema, hypotension and pleural effusions attributed to nonspecific endothelial damage.[4] Patients have developed antibodies not only to murine immunoglobulin, but also to the toxin moieties. Nonetheless, these preliminary studies have demonstrated that immunotoxin can be given with acceptable toxicities. Several transient complete and partial responses have been noted to date,[12,14] which suggests that the immunotoxins have biologic activity in vivo. However, the majority of patients have had bulk and refractory disease. Future studies will evaluate their utility in patients in minimal disease state.

Finally, MoAbs have been conjugated to nuclides in an attempt to enhance cytotoxicity. The most common radionuclides conjugated to MoAbs are the β emitters iodine-131 and yttrium-90; α emitters, such as bismuth-212; and radioisotopes that function by electron capture, such as iodine-125.[4] Most commonly, treated patients include those with hematologic malignancies.[17-19] Of 210 such patients, 19% and 36% achieved complete and partial responses, respectively.[4] The major toxicity of this treatment has been myelosuppression, especially thrombocytopenia.

In-Vitro Use of MoAbs

Bone marrow transplantation (BMT) for patients with leukemia and lymphoma can employ syngeneic, HLA-matched allogeneic or autologous bone marrow grafts. Regardless of the source of the marrow graft, BMT permits escalation of chemotherapeutic drug dose and a multimodality approach, both of which increase the number of complete responses achieved. Studies have demonstrated that high-dose chemotherapy followed by syngeneic or allogeneic BMT can lead to long-term disease-free survival in patients with various hematologic neoplasms, including acute myelogenous leukemia (AML), acute lymphoblastic leukemia (ALL), chronic myelogenous leukemia (CML) and non-Hodgkin's lymphoma (NHL).[20-24] Syngeneic BMT offers the obvious advantages of histocompatibility between donor and recipient and the use of normal marrow, but identical twin donors are available for only a minority of patients. In allogeneic BMT, the donor marrow is also normal, but this approach is limited by graft-vs-host disease (GVHD), even in patients who receive prophylactic regimens, and by the fact that only about 40% of individuals will have HLA-matched marrow donors.[25-31] Most recently, autologous BMT has also proven to be effective treatment for relapsed hematologic malignancies, including AML,[32-36] ALL,[37-40] NHL[24,41-48] and multiple myeloma.[49,50] The major advantage of this approach is the infusion and acceptance of one's own stem and progenitor cells, which eliminates the need for an allogeneic donor and avoids GVHD. The presence of tumor cells in diseases intrinsic to the marrow (ie, leukemia and myeloma) or their high frequency in marrow at the time of relapse (eg, NHL) may limit the utility of this approach. Each marrow source therefore has its potential advantages, but each also has limitations that prevent the more widespread application of this treatment approach.

Monoclonal antibodies have been used to avoid the problems inherent in allogeneic and autologous BMT therapy for hematologic malignancies. Specifically, MoAbs in vitro have been used: 1) to purge tumor cells from marrow prior to autologous BMT[5,32-50] and 2) to deplete donor marrow T lymphocytes to abrogate GVHD in recipients of allogeneic marrow grafts.[5,25-31] As noted above, the initial therapeutic studies of leukemia and lymphoma with MoAbs used in-vivo infusions directed at antigens on the surface of tumor cells, often demonstrated rapid antibody-mediated clearance of tumor cells, but only rarely achieved sustained complete remissions. In-vivo infusions are limited, however, by several problems: delivery of MoAb to the antigen-bearing cell, shedding of cell-surface antigen, antigen-negative tumor cells, the development of blocking antigen or antibody in the host, host reaction to murine immunoglobulins and unexpected MoAb reactivity with host tissues. In contrast, subsequent studies that have used MoAbs in vitro to deplete antigen-bearing target cells from marrow prior to allogeneic and autologous BMT ensure that no blocking antigen or antibody is present, allow close control of culture conditions, ensure that all antigen-bearing cells are in direct contact with MoAb, and allow thorough washing to remove MoAb prior to marrow infusion. Most important, this approach avoids direct exposure of the patient to MoAb, which might result in unexpected reactivity with host tissues and related toxicity.

In-vitro incubation of donor marrow with either single or multiple MoAbs alone does not effectively deplete target cells, however, and various effector systems have been used. The MoAb-based in-vitro methods include MoAb- and complement-mediated lysis, immunotoxins, MoAb-based magnetic, immunoabsorption or MoAb- and pharmacologic-based methodologies to deplete antigen-bearing cells from bone marrow. These in-vitro systems have permitted the exploitation of the specificity of MoAbs to identify well-defined target populations and have vastly increased the spectrum of disease categories and patients who currently may be treated with BMT.

Depletion of Tumor Cells From Autologous Marrow

Autologous BMT after high-dose chemoradiotherapy has achieved 20% to 50% long-term relapse-free survival in patients with high-risk hematologic malignancies or in patients in relapse whose disease remains sensitive to therapy. Most patients with overt tumor in marrow have been excluded from autografting.

The concept of using antibodies and complement to lyse histologically evident tumor cells within autologous bone marrow was initially evaluated with appropriate polyclonal heteroantisera. These early studies were limited by the extensive testing and absorption of antibodies and complement necessary to achieve selective cell kill while preserving hematopoietic cell function.[51] The availability of somatic cell hybridization techniques permitted the development of MoAbs that reacted with normal myeloid and lymphoid cells as well as with a variety of human myeloid and lymphoid malignancies, thereby avoiding problems inherent in heteroantisera. MoAbs have improved specificity, avidity and affinity. As mentioned earlier, studies that have used MoAbs in vitro to lyse antigen-bearing tumor cells from bone marrow ensure that no blocking antigen or antibody is present, allow close control of culture conditions (temperature) to avoid antigen modulation, ensure that all tumor cells are in direct contact with the MoAb, and allow thorough washing to remove the MoAb before marrow infusion. Since most murine MoAbs do not fix human complement, either guinea pig or rabbit complement can be used when lysis of antigen-bearing cells is done in vitro. This MoAb approach also has limitations. First, only murine MoAbs of specific isotypes (IgG2a and IgM) fix complement. Second, the complement source must ensure complete and specific lysis of antigen-bearing cells. Nonetheless, both MoAbs of appropriate isotype and carefully screened xenogenic complement are currently available and have been used under controlled conditions in vitro to ensure specific lysis of residual marrow tumor cells prior to autologous BMT.

The in-vitro culture conditions that must be defined for each MoAb and complement purging technique include the following: optimal MoAb concentration, optimal number of MoAb treatments, optimal bone marrow cell concentration, use of single or multiple MoAbs and the effect of MoAb treatment on normal marrow stem and progenitor cells. Studies of Bast and colleagues[52] provide good examples of this process. They have used [51]chromium-labeled CALLA-positive Nalm 1 cells or lymphoblasts in a 100-fold excess of normal bone marrow cells to demonstrate: 1) that three treatments with anti-CALLA MoAb and complement for 30 minutes was more effective than two treatments for 45 minutes or one treatment for 90 minutes; 2) that concentrations of bone marrow in excess of 2×10^7 cells/mL inhibited treatment with anti-CALLA MoAb and complement; and 3) that repeated treatment with anti-CALLA MoAb and complement, which eliminated more than 99% of the leukemia cells, produced a 50% loss of normal nucleated cells but no selective loss of stem or progenitor cells. In subsequent studies, these investigators have used a clonogenic assay to demonstrate that combinations of two MoAbs were more effective than any single MoAb in eliminating Nalmalwa tumor cells without a concomitant increase in stem cell loss.[53] The combination of multiple MoAbs and 4-hydroperoxycyclophosphamide (4-HC) was significantly more effective than either single agent in removing clonogenic tumor cells. Moreover, Nalmalwa clones resistant to either MoAb or drug treatment were not resistant to the other modality.[54] Other recent studies confirm the utility of combined MoAb and complement plus pharmacologic techniques[34] or of immunomagnetic bead techniques[55] for achieving greater tumor cell depletion than is possible with MoAb and complement alone. These studies are illustrative of those by other investigators who also describe the use of various in-vitro assays to define optimal conditions for and effectiveness of elimination of tumor cells from marrow before autologous BMT for hematologic malignancies. These in-vitro assays also can be used to determine the efficacy of MoAb-based immunomagnetic, immunoadsorption and immunotoxin techniques for the depletion of tumor cells from autologous marrow. The development of these in-vitro assays is essential, for only when a technique that effectively depletes all tumor cells from marrow is defined in vitro can future studies compare autologous BMT using adequately purged versus nonpurged marrows.

A final important requirement for MoAbs that are to be used to purge tumor cells from autologous marrow before autologous BMT is the lack of reactivity with hematopoietic precursors. To date, no assay of marrow graft stem or progenitor cells correlates consistently with engraftment after BMT.[56] Nonetheless, MoAbs are assayed for reactivity with colony-forming units–granulocyte-macrophage (CFU-GM), CFU–granulocyte-erythroid-megakaryocyte-monocyte (CFU-GEMM) or burst-forming units–erythroid before their use for purging autologous marrow. In addition, the effect of a given MoAb treatment on long-term bone marrow cultures can be determined, since these cultures may define an earlier progenitor cell that is closer to the stem cell necessary for sustained hematopoietic engraftment after BMT. Greenberger et al,[57] for example, have established long-term cultures from bone marrow that was treated in vitro with MoAbs to B1 (CD20), J2 (CD9) or J5 (CD10), demonstrating that these antigens are absent on stem cells and suggesting that treatment of marrow with these MoAbs before BMT should not delay or inhibit engraftment. Antibody to the My9 (CD33) antigen, which is present on some CFU-GEMM, does not prevent growth of these long-term marrow cultures. In contrast, treatment of marrow with antibody to Ia and complement kills all detectable cells forming CFU-GEMM, burst-forming units and CFU-GM. In this regard, it has been noted in canine studies that treatment of autologous marrow with Ia MoAb results in complete failure of engraftment and reconstitution after BMT.[58] Thus, all MoAbs under consideration for use in treating marrow before BMT should be screened for their effects on hematopoietic progenitors. The development of stem cell assays that correlate more closely with reconstitution after BMT is also required before the effects of new in-vitro MoAb treatments of marrow can be accurately assessed.

Whether or not tumor cells present in the autologous marrow must be purged before BMT is unknown at this time and may vary, according to the histology and disease status. One might postulate that malignancies that arise from the marrow (eg, leukemias, myelomas) or that are commonly evident within the marrow (eg, relapsed lymphoma) will require purging; however, the need for purging in any setting remains undefined. The limit of histologic detectability of tumor cells is 10^8, and more sensitive techniques such as in-vitro culture, gene rearrangement studies, DNA clonal excess studies and polymerase chain reaction (PCR) techniques permit the detection of tumor cells in marrow without any histologic evidence of malignancy (Fig 7-1). These in-vitro assays may become adaptable, so that an individual patient's marrow may be assayed at the time of bone marrow harvest to define the need for purging. For example, Sharp and coworkers[59] have recently used a culture technique sensitive for detecting occult lymphoma cells in marrow to analyze histologically normal marrow harvested from 59 consecutive patients with intermediate or high-grade NHL who were candidates for high-dose therapy and autologous BMT. Twenty patients had occult lymphoma in their marrow; of the 24 patients who achieved complete remission after BMT, 11 patients with occult

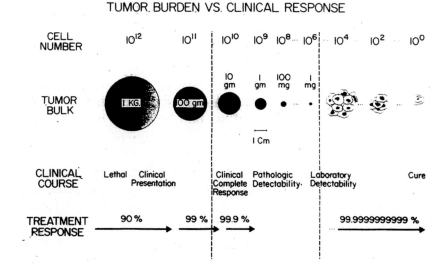

Figure 7-1. Sensitivity of techniques for detection of marrow tumor cells.

lymphoma in their marrow relapsed up to 3 years after transplant, whereas no relapses were observed beyond 8 months in the 13 patients receiving marrow that did not contain detectable lymphoma cells using the culture technique. In this study, detection of lymphoma cells in marrow was an adverse prognostic factor, independent of other clinical features.

In B-cell NHL, PCR techniques have also been used to detect occult tumor cells in autologous marrow grafts on the basis of the tumor specific chromosomal translocation (t14;18), which occurs in 85% of follicular and 30% of diffuse subtypes. For example, PCR has recently demonstrated that immunologic purging using B-cell MoAbs and complement lysis could successfully remove PCR-detectable lymphoma cells from autografts in only half of the patients.[55] Those patients who received autologous marrow containing residual lymphoma cells detectable by PCR had an increased incidence of relapse.[60]

Immunomagnetic bead and complement depletion methods with the same MoAbs achieved 100% and 44% removal of PCR detectable tumor cells,[55] respectively, which suggests that autografting using marrow purged with magnetic bead methodology may achieve superior results. Although there have been several trials of MoAb-purged autografting for patients with AML, the only trials published to date that attempt to correlate clinical outcome with purging used chemotherapeutic (mafosfamide) purging.[33] In that study, 263 patients with AML underwent auto-grafting in first remission: 69 patients received autologous mar-row purged in vitro with mafosfamide; 194 received unpurged marrow. Although that study can be criticized methodologically, it nonetheless reported that patients with standard risk AML in complete remission autografted after cytoreductive regimens containing total-body irradiation had a higher probability of leukemia-free survival and a lower probability of relapse if they received purged rather than unpurged marrow. Chao and col-leagues also suggest that patients with AML who underwent autografting with 4-HC-purged marrow have a longer actuarial disease-free survival and lower relapse rate than similar patients who receive unpurged marrow.[36]

In patients with non-T-cell ALL, Uckun and colleagues[39] have utilized MoAbs and complement coupled with 4-HC purging in an attempt to eliminate residual leukemic cells from autografts prior to BMT. Although these methods depleted $\geq 4 \log_{10}$ of tumor cells in some cases, marked interpatient variability in the effi-ciency of depletion of leukemic progenitor cells was noted, which suggests that improved purging techniques are needed. In preliminary studies utilizing the combination of immunotoxins and 4-HC for in-vitro purging, the number of leukemic progeni-tors remaining in marrow after purging did not correlate with the probability of disease-free survival after BMT. These data suggest that the primary reason for posttransplant recurrence of leukemia was inefficient pretransplant chemotherapy, rather than ineffi-cient purging of autografts.[38] Finally, MoAb- and complement-purged autologous BMT has been compared to allogeneic BMT for patients with refractory, high-risk non-T-cell ALL; this ap-proach can result in 20% long-term relapse-free survival.[40]

In myeloma, MoAb and complement lysis; MoAb and immu-nomagnetic bead; and immunotoxin, pharmacologic or com-bined immunologic- and pharmacologic-based methods have been developed for depleting tumor cells in autografts.[49,61-64] There are no characteristic chromosomal translocations that could be used to identify residual myeloma cells within auto-grafts and assess the efficacy of purging. However, consensus oligonucleotide primers and PCR methodology have recently been used to amplify the third complementary-determining re-gion of rearranged immunoglobulin. Allele-specific oligonu-cleotides derived from the sequences of the PCR products were then used in subsequent amplification reactions to detect malignant clones in the peripheral blood of myeloma patients.[65] Further similar studies will not only allow more precise and quantitative assessment of in-vitro purging techniques, but will also allow for detection of minimal residual disease in vivo after high-dose therapy followed by BMT in patients with myeloma.

Depletion of T Cells From Allogeneic Marrows

Numerous studies have demonstrated that high-dose chemotherapy plus total-body irradiation followed by histocompatible allogeneic BMT can be effective therapy for some patients with AML, ALL, CML and NHL.[20-31] Early studies of HLA-matched allogeneic transplants, which were conducted in patients with relapsed AML refractory to standard chemotherapy, achieved significant tumor cell response and a small (10-20%) percentage of long-term disease-free survivors, but relapse of leukemia occurred in the majority of cases. Subsequent trials of BMT undertaken before leukemia cells had become resistant to standard chemotherapy (ie, in first remission) have achieved actuarial disease-free survival rates at 3 years of 35% to more than 70%, with relapse rates of approximately 25%.[25-31] This is a much lower relapse rate than is noted in patients treated with continued chemotherapy after first remission has been achieved. Direct comparisons, however, of HLA-matched allogeneic BMT in first remission to continued chemotherapy have not yet demonstrated a clear overall survival advantage for either approach because of the early toxicity of BMT. Up to 70% of patients with successful HLA-matched allogeneic marrow grafts will develop GVHD in spite of standard prophylactic therapy to prevent it.[26] If GVHD and posttransplant immunosuppression could be decreased, it is likely that BMT would result in improved survival. Moreover, BMT might then be applicable to older patients. In the setting of unrelated BMT, GVHD occurs in the majority of patients, despite the fact that the marrow donor and recipient are HLA-matched and mixed lymphocyte culture nonreactive.[25] T-cell depletion of the donor marrow has markedly decreased both the incidence and toxicity of GVHD after HLA-matched sibling allografting[28,29,31] and offers similar potential utility in decreasing GVHD after unrelated donor allografting as well.[25] (See also Chapter 9.)

Experimental studies in mice have clearly demonstrated that the major cell responsible for GVHD after allogeneic BMT is a mature

T lymphocyte and that GVHD can be prevented if these T cells are eliminated from the donor marrow before transplantation. T-cell removal has been accomplished by means of heterologous antisera specific for T cells plus complement, antibody-toxin conjugates or lectin agglutination. In these experiments, GVHD was completely prevented, thereby allowing transplantation and reconstitution across major histocompatibility barriers. In analogous human studies, T cells have been removed from allogeneic marrow prior to BMT using E rosette and lectin agglutination, counterflow centrifugation elutriation, MoAb- and complement-mediated lysis, MoAb bound to toxin, and MoAb-based magnetic and MoAb-based immunoadsorption techniques, but not by incubation of marrow with either single or multiple T-cell MoAbs alone.[5,28,29,31] The effectiveness of depleting T cells in allogeneic marrow has been assessed both by limiting dilution assays and by functional analysis of treated marrow for residual T cells. In both animal and human studies, various techniques for the depletion of donor marrow T cells prior to allogeneic BMT have significantly decreased the incidence and severity of GVHD.

A potential advantage of using MoAb-depletion techniques is the ability to remove only those T cells expressing specific T-cell surface antigens (Fig 7-2). Anti T-12 (CD6), for example, depletes only mature T cells in contrast to E rosette, lectin depletion or elutriation, which may remove all T subsets and some non-T cells. The specificity of MoAbs may potentially avoid the graft rejection and/or graft failure that have been noted in studies of T-cell-depleted marrow.[66] If the T-cell-depleted graft is more easily rejected by the host than a non-T-cell depleted graft, two remedies could be attempted. The first is to use the specificity of MoAbs to deplete a more restricted population of T cells from the donor marrow; the second is to use additional immunosuppressive therapy of the host. Alternatively, if T-cell-depleted marrows fail to engraft, MoAbs could potentially be useful to define those T cells, if any, that are necessary for engraftment. MoAb-based techniques could then be used to specifically deplete all marrow T cells except those cells that are required for engraftment. A further potential advantage of the restricted reactivity of MoAbs may be the definition of those cells that mediate GVHD versus those that mediate the graft-vs-leukemia (GVL) effect. As noted previously, GVHD is mediated by alloreactive T cells, but the cells responsible for GVL effect have not been defined and may be either a subset of T cells or of natural killer

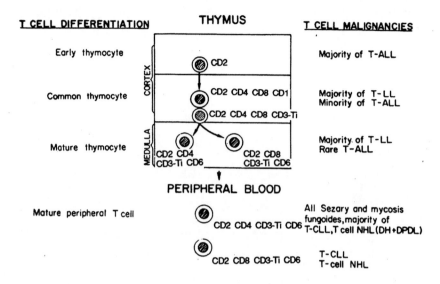

Figure 7-2. Stages of normal and malignant T-cell differentiation.

cells. MoAb-based T-cell-depletion techniques that deplete cells mediating GVHD but preserve those effecting a GVL reaction might then be employed both to avoid GVHD and to prolong long-term engraftment and disease-free survival.

Recently 112 consecutive adult patients with hematologic malignancies were treated with high-dose therapy followed by HLA-matched sibling BMT.[31] Selective in-vitro T-cell depletion with anti-T12 (CD6) MoAb reduced the incidence of both acute and chronic GVHD after allogeneic BMT, without compromising engraftment. Moreover, depletion of CD6-positive cells from marrow obviates the need to administer posttransplant immunosuppression for GVHD prophylaxis to the majority of patients. Thus, the development of T-cell MoAbs that specifically define biologically important subsets of T cells may make BMT a much safer therapy for patients who have histocompatible donors. It may also facilitate the use of HLA-incompatible donors for patients who would not otherwise be candidates for allogeneic BMT.

Future Directions

Autologous hematopoietic stem cell transplantation permits the use of high-dose chemoradiotherapeutic treatments for patients

· with incurable malignancies, as well as for patients with diseases responsive to allogeneic BMT who lack appropriately matched sibling or unrelated donors. Although the need for purging of autologous marrow prior to autografting is at present undefined, sensitive methods are currently available both for evaluating the efficiency of in-vitro purging techniques and for assessment of minimal residual disease after transplantation. These technologies will facilitate development of optimal purging techniques and then allow future randomized studies of purged vs non-purged marrow autografting to establish its value. They will also permit determination of the efficacy and clinical value of various techniques for depleting T cells from marrow prior to allogeneic marrow transplantation. The blood component laboratory has expertise in collection, processing, quality control, cryopreservation, and thawing of cellular blood components for procedures that are essential if marrow grafting is to be successful. Transfusion medicine expertise will, therefore, remain central to and critical in all aspects of hematopoietic stem cell transplantation, both in current practice and in furthering research efforts.[67]

References

1. Anderson KC, Bates MP, Slaughenhoupt BL, et al. Expression of human B cell-associated antigens on leukemias and lymphomas: A model of human B cell differentiation. Blood 1984;63:1424-33.
2. Nadler LM, Korsmeyer SJ, Anderson KC, et al. B cell origin of non-T cell acute lymphoblastic leukemia: A model for discrete stages of neoplastic and normal pre-B cell differentiation. J Clin Invest 1984;74:332-40.
3. Anderson KC, Boyd AW, Fisher DC, et al. Hairy cell leukemia: A tumor of pre-plasma cells. Blood 1985;65:620-9.
4. Grossbard ML, Press OW, Appelbaum FR, et al. Monoclonal antibody-based therapies of leukemia and lymphoma. Blood 1992;80:863-78.
5. Anderson KC, Nadler LM, Takvorian T, et al. Monoclonal antibodies: Their use in bone marrow transplantation. In: Brown E, ed. Progress in hematology. Orlando: Grune and Stratton, 1987:137-81.
6. Klein B, Wijdenes J, Zhang X-G, et al. Murine anti-interleukin-6 monoclonal antibody therapy for a patient with plasma cell leukemia. Blood 1991;78:1198-204.

7. Anderson KC, Jones RM, Morimoto C, et al. Response patterns of purified myeloma cells to hematopoietic growth factors. Blood 1989;73:1915-24.

8. Dillman RO, Beauregard JC, Halpern SE, Clutter M. Toxicities and side effects associated with intravenous infusions of murine monoclonal antibodies. J Biol Response Mod 1986;5:73-84.

9. Brown SL, Miller RA, Horning SJ, et al. Treatment of B-cell lymphomas with anti-idiotype antibodies alone and in combination with alpha interferon. Blood 1989;73:651-61.

10. Waldmann TA, Goldman CK, Bongiovanni KF, et al. Therapy of patients with human T-cell lymphotrophic virus I-induced adult T-cell leukemia with anti-Tac, a monoclonal antibody to the receptor for interleukin-2. Blood 1988;72:1805-16.

11. Endo Y, Mitsui K, Motizuki M, Tsurugi K. The mechanism of action of ricin and related toxic lectins on eukaryotic ribosomes. J Biol Chem 1987;262:5908-12.

12. Grossbard ML, Freedman AS, Ritz J, et al. Serotherapy of B-cell neoplasms with anti-B4-blocked ricin: A phase I trial of bolus infusion. Blood 1992;79:576-85.

13. Collier RJ. Effect of diphtheria toxin on protein synthesis: Inactivation of one of the transfer factors. J Mol Biol 1967;25:83-98.

14. LeMaistre CF, Meneghetti C, Rosenblum M, et al. Phase I trial of interleukin-2 (IL-2) fusion toxin ($DAB_{486}IL-2$) in hematologic malignancies expressing the IL-2 receptor. Blood 1992;79:2547-54.

15. Hwang J, Fitzgerald DJ, Adhya S, Pastan I. Functional domains of Pseudomonas exotoxin identified by deletion analysis of the gene expressed in *E. coli*. Cell 1987;48:129-36.

16. Kreitman RJ, Siegall CB, Fitzgerald DJP, et al. Interleukin-6 fused to a mutant form of Pseudomonas exotoxin kills malignant cells from patients with multiple myeloma. Blood 1993;79:1775-80.

17. Press OW, Eary JF, Badger CC, et al. Treatment of refractory non-Hodgkin's lymphoma with radiolabeled MB-1 (anti-CD37) antibody. J Clin Oncol 1989;7:1027-38.

18. Goldenberg DM, Horowitz JA, Sharkey RM, et al. Targeting, dosimetry, and radioimmunotherapy of B-cell lymphomas with iodine-131-labeled LL2 monoclonal antibody. J Clin Oncol 1991;9:548-64.

19. Vriesendorp HM, Herpst JM, Germack MA, et al. Phase I-II studies of yttrium-labeled antiferritin treatment for end-stage Hodgkin's disease, including Radiation Therapy Oncology Group 87-01. J Clin Oncol 1991;9:918-28.

20. Blaise D, Maraninchi E, Archimbaud E, et al. Allogeneic bone marrow transplantation for acute myeloid leukemia in first remission: A randomized trial of a busulfan-cytoxan versus cytoxan-total body irradiation as preparative regimen: A Report from the Groupe d'Études de la Greffe de Moelle Osseuse. Blood 1992;79:2578-82.

21. Ramsay NKC, Kersey JH. Indications for marrow transplantation in acute lymphoblastic leukemia. Blood 1990;75:815-18.

22. Delage R, Ritz J, Anderson KC. The evolving role of bone marrow transplantation in the treatment of chronic myelogenous leukemia. Hematol Oncol Clin North Am 1990;4:369-88.

23. Anderson KC, Nadler LM. Bone marrow transplantation in the therapy of non-Hodgkin's lymphoma. In: DeVita VT Jr, Hellman S, Rosenberg SA, eds. Important advances in oncology. Philadelphia: JB Lippincott, 1986:287-310.

24. Armitage JO. Bone marrow transplantation in the treatment of patients with lymphoma. Blood 1989;73:1749-58.

25. Ash RC, Casper JT, Christopher R, et al. Successful allogeneic transplantation of T-cell-depleted bone marrow from closely HLA-matched unrelated donors. N Engl J Med 1990;8:485-94.

26. Atkinson K, Horowitz MM, Gale RP, et al. Risk factors for chronic graft-versus-host disease after HLA-identical sibling bone marrow transplantation. Blood 1990;75:2459-64.

27. Martin PJ, Schoch G, Fisher L, et al. A retrospective analysis of therapy for acute graft-versus-host disease: Initial treatment. Blood 1990;76:1464-72.

28. Champlin R, Ho W, Gajewski J, et al. Selective depletion of CD8+T lymphocytes for prevention of graft-versus-host-disease after allogeneic bone marrow transplantation. Blood 1990;76:418-23.

29. Marmont AM, Horowitz MM, Gale RP et al. T-cell depletion of HLA-identical transplants in leukemia. Blood 1991;78:2120-30.

30. Nash RA, Pepe MS, Storb R, et al. Acute graft-versus-host disease: Analysis of risk factors after allogeneic marrow

transplantation and prophylaxis with cyclosporine and methotrexate. Blood 1992;80:1838-45.

31. Soiffer RJ, Murray C, Mauch P, et al. Prevention of graft-versus-host disease by selective depletion of CD6-positive T lymphocytes from donor bone marrow. J Clin Oncol 1992;10:1191-200.

32. Ball ED, Mills LE, Cornwell GG III, et al. Autologous bone marrow transplantation for acute myeloid leukemia using monoclonal antibody-purged bone marrow. Blood 1990;75:1199-206.

33. Gorin NC, Aegerter P, Auvert B, et al. Autologous bone marrow transplantation for acute myelocytic leukemia in first remission: A European survey of the role of marrow purging. Blood 1990;75:1606-14.

34. Lemoli RM, Gasparetto C, Scheinberg DA, et al. Autologous bone marrow transplantation in acute myelogenous leukemia: In vitro treatment with myeloid-specific monoclonal antibodies and drugs in combination. Blood 1991;77:1829-36.

35. Robertson MJ, Soiffer RJ, Freedman AS, et al. Human bone marrow depleted of CD33-positive cells mediates delayed but durable reconstitution of hematopoiesis: Clinical trial of MY9 monoclonal antibody-purged autografts for the treatment of acute myeloid leukemia. Blood 1992;79:2229-36.

36. Chao NJ, Stein AS, Long GD, et al. Busulfan/etoposide—Initial experience with a new preparatory regimen for autologous bone marrow transplantation in patients with acute nonlymphoblastic leukemia. Blood 1993;81:319-23.

37. Sallan SE, Niemeyer CM, Billett AL, et al. Autologous bone marrow transplantation for acute lymphoblastic leukemia. J Clin Oncol 1989;7:1594-601.

38. Uckun FM, Kersey JH, Vallera DA, et al. Autologous bone marrow transplantation in high-risk remission T-lineage acute lymphoblastic leukemia using immunotoxins plus 4-hydroperoxycyclophosphamide for marrow purging. Blood 1990;76:1723-33.

39. Uckun FM, Kersey JH, Haake R, et al. Autologous bone marrow transplantation in high-risk remission B-lineage acute lymphoblastic leukemia using a cocktail of three monoclonal antibodies (BA-1/CD24, BA-2/CD9, and BA-3/CD10) plus complement and 4-hydroperoxycyclophos-

phamide for ex vivo bone marrow purging. Blood 1992;79:1094-104.

40. Kersey JH, Weisdorf D, Nesbit ME, et al. Comparison of autologous and allogeneic bone marrow transplantation for treatment of high-risk refractory acute lymphoblastic leukemias. N Engl J Med 1987;317:461-7.

41. Takvorian T, Canellos GP, Ritz J, et al. Prolonged disease-free survival after autologous bone marrow transplantation in patients with non-Hodgkin's lymphoma with a poor prognosis. N Engl J Med 1987;316:1499-505.

42. Philip T, Armitage JO, Spitzer G, et al. High-dose therapy and autologous bone marrow transplantation after failure of conventional chemotherapy in adults with intermediate-grade or high-grade non-Hodgkin's lymphoma. N Engl J Med 1987;316:1493-8.

43. Hurd DD, LeBien TW, Lasky LC, et al. Autologous bone marrow transplantation in non-Hodgkin's lymphoma: Monoclonal antibodies plus complement for ex vivo marrow treatment. Am J Med 1988;85:829-34.

44. Freedman AS, Takvorian T, Anderson KC, et al. Autologous bone marrow transplantation in B-cell non-Hodgkin's lymphoma: Very low treatment-related mortality in 100 patients in sensitive relapse. J Clin Oncol 1990;8:784-91.

45. Anderson KC, Soiffer R, DeLage R, et al. T-cell-depleted autologous bone marrow transplantation therapy: Analysis of immune deficiency and late complications. Blood 1990;76:235-44.

46. Freedman AS, Ritz J, Neuberg D, et al. Autologous bone marrow transplantation in 69 patients with a history of low-grade B-cell non-Hodgkin's lymphoma. Blood 1991;77:2524-9.

47. Nademanee A, Schmidt GM, O'Donnell MR, et al. High-dose chemoradiotherapy followed by autologous bone marrow transplantation as consolidation therapy during first complete remission in adult patients with poor-risk aggressive lymphoma: A pilot study. Blood 1992;80:1130-4.

48. Gorin NC, Coiffier B, Hayat M, et al. Recombinant human granulocyte-macrophage colony-stimulating factor after high-dose chemotherapy and autologous bone marrow transplantation with unpurged and purged marrow in non-Hodgkin's lymphoma: A double-blind placebo-controlled trial. Blood 1992;80;1149-57.

49. Anderson KC, Barut BA, Ritz J, et al. Monoclonal antibody-purged autologous bone marrow transplantation therapy for multiple myeloma. Blood 1991;77:712-20.

50. Barlogie B, Gahrton G. Bone marrow transplantation in multiple myeloma. Bone Marrow Transplant 1991;7:71-9.

51. Feeney MJ, Knapp RC, Greenberger JS, Bast RC Jr. Elimination of leukemic cells from rat bone marrow using antibody and complement. Cancer Res 1981;41:3331-5.

52. Bast RC Jr, Ritz J, Lipton JM, et al. Elimination of leukemic cells from human bone marrow using monoclonal antibody and complement. Cancer Res 1983;43:1389-94.

53. Bast RC Jr, DeFabritiis P, Lipton J, et al. Elimination of malignant clonogenic cells from human bone marrow using multiple monoclonal antibodies and complement. Cancer Res 1985;45:499-503.

54. DeFabritiis P, Bregni M, Lipton J, et al. Elimination of clonogenic Burkitt's lymphoma cells from human bone marrow using 4-hydroperoxycyclophosphamide in combination with monoclonal antibodies and complement. Blood 1985;65:1064-70.

55. Gribben JG, Saporito L, Barber M, et al. Bone marrows of non-Hodgkin's lymphoma patients with a bcl-2 translocation can be purged of polymerase chain reaction-detectable lymphoma cells using monoclonal antibodies and immunomagnetic bead depletion. Blood 1992;80;1083-9.

56. Atkinson K, Norrie S, Chan P, et al. Lack of correlation between nucleated bone marrow cell dose, marrow CFU-GM dose, marrow CFU-E dose, and the rate of HLA-identical sibling marrow engraftment. Br J Haematol 1985;60:245-51.

57. Greenberger JS, Rothstein L, DeFabritiis P, et al. Effects of monoclonal antibody and complement treatment of human marrow on hematopoiesis in continuous bone marrow culture. Cancer Res 1985;45:758-67.

58. Szer J, Deeg HJ, Appelbaum FR, Storb R. Failure of autologous bone marrow reconstitution after cytolytic treatment of marrow with anti-Ia monoclonal antibody. Blood 1985;65:819-22.

59. Sharp JG, Joshi SS, Armitage JO, et al. Significance of detection of occult non-Hodgkin's lymphoma in histologically uninvolved bone marrow by a culture technique. Blood 1992;79:1074-80.

60. Gribben JG, Freedman AS, Neuberg D, et al. Immunologic purging of marrow assessed by PCR before autologous bone marrow transplantation for B-cell lymphoma. N Engl J Med 1991;325:1525-33.
61. Tong AW, Lee JC, Fay JW, Stone MJ. Elimination of clonogenic stem cells from human multiple myeloma cell lines by a plasma cell-reactive monoclonal antibody and complement. Blood 1987;70:1482-9.
62. Kulkarni SS, Wang Z, Spitzer G, et al. Elimination of drug-resistant myeloma tumor cell lines by monoclonal anti-P-glycoprotein antibody and rabbit complement. Blood 1989;74:2244-51.
63. Shimazaki C, Wisniewski D, Scheinberg DA, et al. Elimination of myeloma cells from bone marrow by using monoclonal antibodies and magnetic immunobeads. Blood 1988;72:1248-54.
64. Rhodes EGH, Baker PK, Duguid JKM, et al. A method for clinical purging of myeloma bone marrow using peanut agglutinin as an anti-plasma cell agent, in combination with CD19 monoclonal antibody. Bone Marrow Transplant 1992;10:485-9.
65. Billadeau D, Quam L, Thomas W, et al. Detection and quantitation of malignant cells in the peripheral blood of multiple myeloma patients. Blood 1992;80:1818-24.
66. Goldman JM, Gale RP, Horowitz MM, et al. Bone marrow transplantation for chronic myelogenous leukemia in chronic phase: Increased risk for relapse associated with T-cell depletion. Ann Intern Med 1988;108:806-14.
67. Anderson KC. The role of the blood bank in hematopoietic stem cell transplantation. Transfusion 1992;32:272-85.

In: Lasky L and Warkentin P, eds. *Marrow and Stem Cell Processing for Transplantation*
Bethesda, MD: American Association of Blood Banks, 1995

8

Pharmacologic Purging of Bone Marrow

Scott D. Rowley, MD, FACP

AUTOLOGOUS BONE MARROW TRANSPLANTATION (BMT) allows the use of high-dose "marrow-lethal" chemotherapy or radiotherapy regimens in the treatment of dose-responsive cancers. These regimens, used for diseases in which a small increase in the intensity of the regimen may result in greatly increased efficacy of tumor kill, require transfusion of cells from a healthy donor to rescue the patient from prolonged and probably fatal aplasia. An alternative to transplantation of hematopoietic progenitor cells from a healthy donor is the storage of adequate numbers of progenitor cells harvested from the patient before the conditioning regimen is initiated. In theory, however, the harvested marrow cells may be contaminated with occult tumor cells [minimal residual disease (MRD)] that are not evident during the preharvest evaluation of the patient. Cancers of the bone marrow such as acute leukemia or multiple myeloma are presumed to contain malignant stem cells capable of causing relapse after infusion into the patient. Other cancers such as lymphoma or breast cancer frequently involve the bone marrow at some point during the natural history of the disease. In an attempt to remove MRD and improve the probability of successful transplant outcome, several transplant centers developed and studied techniques to remove, or purge, the malignant cells from the marrow after harvesting, while preserving the normal hematopoietic cells required for hematologic recovery from the conditioning regimen.

A number of purging techniques have been developed. All techniques must be capable of discriminating between the malignant and the normal precursors in the bone marrow. For some

Scott D. Rowley, MD, FACP, Associate Member, Fred Hutchinson Cancer Research Center, Director, Clinical Cryobiology Laboratory, Seattle, Washington diseases, cell surface antigens present on the tumor cell but not on the hematopoietic stem cell can be exploited for separation. Murine monoclonal antibodies are highly selective and when combined with complement, toxin molecules or physical separation, can achieve very efficient depletion of the tumor cells. These immunologic techniques have been widely employed in the treatment of lymphoid malignancies such as non-Hodgkin's lymphoma (NHL) or acute lymphoblastic leukemia (ALL). The development of antibodies against acute myelocytic leukemic cells was more difficult because these cells share antigens present on normal hematopoietic cells. Thus, immunologic purging in this disease does not achieve the high degree of selectivity found in treating lymphoid (or other nonmyeloid) malignancies. In addition, immunologic techniques may be of limited efficacy because of tumor cell heterogeneity (requiring multiple antibodies directed against different cell surface antigens for greatest effect). In contrast, pharmacologic agents that are sparing of hematopoietic stem cells may be useful for ex-vivo purging of a wide variety of malignancies, although the sensitivity of the malignancy to the drug(s) must be determined first. The requirements of a purging agent, whether it be immunologic or pharmacologic, are 1) that the agent spare the hematopoietic cells necessary for hematologic recovery after high-dose therapy, 2) that the agent be very effective in the killing of tumor cells during the brief exposure usually available before cryopreservation and 3) that the agent be removable, or be nontoxic upon transfusion of the bone marrow cells to the patient. Inherent to these properties are that the agent be able to kill malignant cells regardless of cell cycle status, and that drug levels be several times higher than those achievable in vivo. Initial preclinical studies demonstrated the feasibility of treating hematopoietic cells with pharmacologics. Subsequent Phase I and II clinical trials established that bone marrow cells could be treated ex vivo with drug concentrations not achievable in vivo and still allow engraftment.

Rationale for Purging

The initial rationale for purging harvested cells was based upon the natural history of the cancers being treated. For acute leukemia or multiple myeloma, which are malignancies of the bone marrow, it is expected that malignant cells will be harvested along with the normal cells. Such diseases as breast cancer or lymphoma frequently metastasize to the bone marrow at some point during the natural history of the disease. For other malignancies such as Hodgkin's disease, ovarian cancer or glioblastoma, bone marrow involvement is much rarer. Thus, patients undergoing autologous BMT for acute leukemia, for example, could be expected to benefit from purging of the bone marrow. (This argument presumes that the patient is not cured of malignancy before undergoing the marrow harvest.)

Numerical arguments have been proffered supporting or negating the necessity of purging for optimal disease-free survival after autologous transplantation. The first simply states that, by definition, a remission bone marrow for patients with acute myelogenous leukemia (AML) may contain up to 5% blasts, and therefore, the average harvest of 3×10^8 cells/kg of patient weight for a 70-kg patient (2.1×10^{10} cells) could contain up to 1×10^8 tumor cells. Thus, an ideal purging agent, whether immunologic or pharmacologic, must be capable of depleting "8 $\log_{10}$" of tumor cells. This is especially important for patients with AML in second or subsequent remission where the chances are very low that the patient's marrow will be free of disease at the time of harvest. One reasonable, but theoretical argument against purging is based upon the presumed characteristics of the malignant cell and its cryosurvival (Table 8-1).[1] The authors of this argument proposed that not all malignant cells identifiable by microscopy are

Table 8-1. Numerical Argument Against Purging Efficacy for AML

Time Point	Effect	Number of Leukemic Cells*
Diagnosis		10^{13} per patient
Remission induction	Deplete 10^4 leukemic cells	10^9 per patient
Marrow harvest	Collect 1.5% of marrow cells	1.5×10^6 per graft
Cryopreservation	1% survival of AML cells	1.5×10^4 per graft
Infusion	0.1-1% of AML cells are clonal	15-150 clonal tumor cells infused

*Shown are the number of leukemic cells in the patient or the portion of bone marrow cells harvested for autologous bone marrow transplantation at various time points after diagnosis and during therapy. (Adapted from Schultz FW, et al.[1])

capable of clonal growth and causing relapse after infusion (and thus, 8 $\log_{10}$ of purging is not required). They also suggested that the malignant cell poorly tolerates cryopreservation.[2] Finally, the number of clonogenic cells required to cause relapse after infusion is not known, but it is almost certainly more than one. Thus, the "in-vitro" purging achieved by the preharvest chemotherapy, coupled with cryopreservation damage and the presumed nonuniform clonality of the malignant cell population, may negate the need for ex-vivo purging of the harvested bone marrow. These considerations may apply to other malignancies as well, and proof of purging efficacy for one disease cannot be extended to others.

These theoretical arguments regarding purging in the treatment of AML are now of historical interest only. Although it is reasonable to expect that multiple courses of chemotherapy before marrow harvesting may reduce the level of malignant cells below a critical threshold for causing subsequent relapse, recent experiments have demonstrated the capacity of leukemic cells in the marrow inoculum to contribute to relapse after autologous BMT.[3] Brenner and colleagues harvested bone marrow from patients with acute myelocytic leukemia in first remission, marked a portion of the cells with a DNA fragment encoding neomycin resistance and cryopreserved the cells without purging. Of 10 patients who underwent transplantation with the marked marrows, two have relapsed and leukemic blasts from both showed the neomycin resistance gene previously inserted. This experiment does not prove that the harvested bone marrow was the sole source for relapse after transplantation, but it does suggest that some form of ex-vivo purging, or more extensive preharvest chemotherapy ("in-vitro purging"), may be necessary for optimal results after autologous BMT for this disease for selected patients. Similar studies have not been reported for other malignancies. Anecdotal reports of miliary relapses after autologous BMT cannot be used to support the need for purging for breast cancer, NHL or other cancers because such widespread involvement may result from the immune suppression of the high-dose chemotherapy given, with uncontrolled growth of residual tumor in the patient, and not from transfusion of malignant cells in the marrow inoculum.

As noted above, purging cannot be justified for diseases that do not involve the bone marrow, no matter how minimal the perceived risk or cost to the patient. No manipulation of marrow is free of risk. Ideally, techniques that assess the quantity of tumor contamination will be developed to allow purging to be limited to those patients who would most benefit from this therapy. In the absence of such techniques, purging should be limited to defined populations of patients who have been shown to benefit from this therapy.

Rationale for Pharmacologic Purging

Chemotherapeutics offer defined advantages for purging of malignant cells. Compared to monoclonal antibodies that are very specific in the type of cell that may be removed, pharmacologic agents show a broad range of activity. Even tumors that are not considered sensitive to a particular drug administered directly to the patient may be effectively depleted when exposed to the very high concentrations frequently tolerated by hematopoietic progenitor cells in vitro. Bone marrow transplantation is most effective in dose-responsive malignancies in which escalation of the drugs may achieve much greater tumor cell kill and cure of the disease. The greater escalation of drug dosage during the in-vitro marrow treatment would, therefore, also be expected to result in considerable tumor cell kill. Combinations of drugs may be synergistic in killing tumor cells. Finally, pharmaceutics are generally more available and less costly to use than monoclonal antibodies.

Preclinical Evaluation of Pharmacologic Purging Agents

The same principles that apply to the systemic treatment of cancer with chemotherapeutics also apply to their use as ex-vivo purge agents. Dose, duration of exposure, drug metabolism, sensitivity patterns of normal and malignant cells, and mechanisms of cytotoxicity and resistance must all be considered in developing either systemic or ex-vivo regimens. Some drugs such as vincristine or cytosine arabinoside are cycle-specific, killing cells only during certain phases of the cell cycle. These drugs may not be ideal for purging of bone marrow cells because of the brief period usually available before the marrow cells must be cryopreserved. For this reason, alkylating agents, which are cycle-nonspecific, may achieve more effective cytotoxicity against the entire population of malignant cells in the bone marrow inoculum.

A number of drugs have been tested in preclinical assays using tumor-derived cells lines and hematopoietic progenitors cultured from healthy bone marrow donors (Table 8-2).[4-7] These studies are important for demonstrating the potential activity of the agents under study. For example, L-asparaginase would probably not be an active agent. Such studies are also valuable for initial approximation of incubation temperature, duration and cell concentration. In contrast, dose and efficacy can only be determined in clinical trials. The limitation of these preclinical experiments is that derived tumor cell lines may show different patterns of sensitivity than fresh tumor. Furthermore, different cell lines may show different sensitivities to the same agent.

Similarly, progenitor cells that can be cultured in vitro are not the hematopoietic stem cells responsible for long-term engraftment after bone marrow transplantation. Such cultures may be of value in developing incubation parameters. For example, in-vitro cultures assisted in the change to incubating light-density cells rather than buffy-coat cells with 4-hydroperoxycyclophosphamide (4-HC) without requiring a Phase I dose-finding trial.[9] These cultures are of greatest value when a correlation between progenitor cells and engraftment can be demonstrated.

At present, it is much simpler to study the in-vitro cytotoxic effects of drugs than to demonstrate efficacy and safety in clinical trials. In-vitro studies using derived cell lines can be completed in weeks rather than the months to years required for clinical

Table 8-2. Preclinical Evaluation of Drug Purging Agents

Drug*	Cell Line Kill[†] %	CFU-GM Kill %	References
4-HC	83->99.9[a,b,c,d]	82.5-98.8	4,5,6,7
VP16	96.1->99.9[a,c,d]	72.7-97	5,6,7
Vincristine	75->99.9[b,c,d]	<10-76	4,6,7
Adriamycin	98.6->99.3[a,c]	50.6-83	5,6
Bleomycin	19->91.6[b,c]	50-83.5	4,6
L-Asparaginase	0[b]	73.5	4
Cisplatinum	>99.9[c]	96	6

* Drug concentrations, cell concentrations, and incubation durations differ for the various studies.
† Cell lines tested: a) HL-60; b) REH, KM3, LAZ 221; c) LY-16, SK-DHL-2; d) K562, CEM, REH.
(Reprinted with permission from Rowley.[8])

studies. Relatively few drugs have been studied in clinical toxicity or efficacy studies. Cyclophosphamide derivatives have been
the most extensively studied, because of the relative sparing of
hematopoietic stem cells by this agent. The value of these preclinical studies is that they allow the selection of agents that may
be effective in clinical trials and the determination of the initial
treatment parameters.

Purging With Activated Oxazaphosphorines

Pharmacology

4-HC and mafosfamide are activated oxazaphosphorines, derivatives of cyclophosphamide that do not require hepatic metabo-

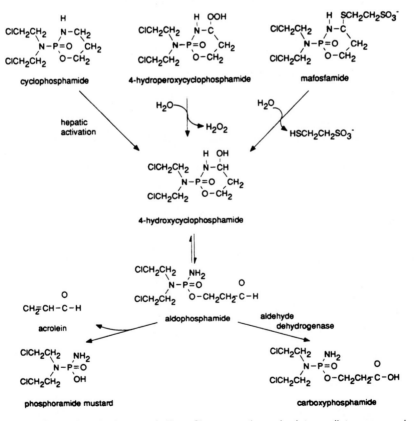

Figure 8-1. Oxazaphosphorine metabolism. Shown are the major intermediate compounds
and metabolic pathways for cyclophosphamide, 4-hydroperoxycyclophosphamide, and mafosfamide.[10] (Reprinted by permission of Blackwell Scientific Publications, Inc.[8])

lism for activity (Fig 8-1).[10] Both 4-HC and mafosfamide spontaneously decompose to 4-hydroxycyclophosphamide in the presence of water. 4-Hydroxycyclophosphamide and aldophosphamide freely penetrate the cell, where activation to phosphoramide mustard or enzymatic oxidation to the inactive metabolite, carboxyphosphamide, occurs. For all three drugs, phosphoramide mustard is the active metabolite. The relative resistance of normal hematopoietic progenitor cells compared to malignant cells, and of mature compared to more primitive stem cells, probably results from differing cellular levels of aldehyde dehydrogenase.[11-16] Hematopoietic stem cells are relatively protected by their increased levels of this enzyme and ability to rapidly degrade the intermediate compounds. Peripheral blood cells also contain aldehyde dehydrogenase and comprise the largest fraction of cells in the incubation mixture. Thus, variation in the cellular content of the incubation mixture (eg, red blood cell content) can result in variations in 4-HC cytotoxicity to both normal and malignant cells, affecting the duration of posttransplant aplasia and, possibly, the risk of relapse after transplantation.[17-19]

Preclinical Studies

The feasibility of pharmacologic purging was demonstrated by Sharkis et al using a rat model of leukemia.[20] They seeded leukemic cells into rat bone marrow, and then purged the mixture with increasing concentrations of 4-HC. They showed that 4-HC was able to prevent the development of leukemia by the recipient of the treated marrow cells, but did not prevent recovery of the rat from the lethal dose of irradiation used to condition the rats for transplantation. At low concentrations of 4-HC, the transplanted animals died of leukemia. The time to death was prolonged as compared to that for animals receiving untreated mixtures of cells. At higher concentrations, the animals survived without leukemia. Thus, 4-HC killed the leukemic cells, but spared the normal cells responsible for hematologic recovery.

Clinical Trials

Investigators at Johns Hopkins University (Baltimore, MD) subsequently performed a Phase I trial of 4-HC purging for patients with AML, ALL, or NHL.[21] The endpoint of this study was engraftment within 3 or 4 weeks after marrow infusion. At the level of 120 µg/mL of 4-HC, several patients did not recover hematopoietic function within this time. Therefore, these investigators defined the maximally tolerated dose for 4-HC as 100 µg/mL. They had no in-vitro measure of 4-HC cytotoxicity to the normal hematopoietic progenitors. This dose was determined from the observed delay in hematologic engraftment. A number of Phase II studies, mostly of patients with AML, were subsequently reported from various transplant centers (Table 8-3).[21-25]

Similar concentrations (µg/mL) of mafosfamide and 4-HC were used in many of the clinical studies, but, because of the higher molecular weight of mafosfamide, the molarity of this drug in the incubation mixture was less. Differences may exist in the rates of initial breakdown to 4-hydroxycyclophosphamide after addition of water. Thus, strict comparison of 4-HC and mafosfamide cytotoxicity is difficult.

The purging technique used by most transplant centers involved treatment of bone marrow buffy-coat cells isolated by centrifugation. The cells were incubated with freshly dissolved 4-HC at 100 µg/mL for 30 minutes at 37 C, followed by chilling to 4 C, decanting of the supernatant fluid and cryopreservation. This technique was modified after the effect of variable red blood cell (and nucleated cell) content of the incubation mixture was found in modulating the cytotoxicity achieved.[17-19] Virtually all current clinical studies limit the red blood cell concentration to between 5-10%. However, limiting the allowable range for the red blood cell concentration in the incubation mixture may poorly regulate the concentration of cellular aldehyde dehydrogenase, an intracellular enzyme responsible for the inactivation of aldophosphamide (Fig 8-1), because the concentration of this enzyme in the blood cells of different patients may differ. It is possible to separate light-density cells before 4-HC incubation, thereby eliminating almost all red blood cells. The concentration of 4-HC must be reduced in response to the decreased inactivation of the drug, although it appears that incubation of density-gradient-separated cells results in less patient-to-patient variability in 4-HC cytotoxicity.[9]

Efficacy

Despite the large numbers of patients treated to date with 4-HC, the efficacy of this drug (and other purging techniques) has not been shown in Phase III studies. The evidence supporting effi-

Table 8-3. Phase II Trials of Activated Oxazaphosphorine Purging for Acute Leukemia

Center*	Diagnosis	No. Patients	CFU-GM Survival Median (Range)	Median Days to:			EFS	Reference
				Granulocytes >500/μL	Platelets >50 K/μL			
Baltimore	AML	25	ND[†]	29	57		43%	21
Pittsburgh	AML	24	0.3% (0-36)	30	91		19%	22
Los Angeles	AML	13	0% (0-3)	40	58		61%	23
Paris	AML, ALL	24	2% (0-47)	ND[†]	67		27-72%[‡]	22
Heidelberg	AML	52	17% (2-100)	29	ND[†]		45%	25

* Marrows treated by the Paris and Heidelberg transplant programs were treated with mafosfamide. The other centers used 4-HC. Light-density marrow cells were isolated before drug treatment by density-gradient separation over Ficoll-Metrizoate (Heidelberg) or a combination gradient of Ficoll-Hypaque layered over Percoll (Los Angeles).
† This particular parameter was not specified in the report.
‡ Patients were classified into high- and low-risk groups, as defined by the authors.

cacy is limited: First, it may be argued that the event-free survival (EFS, censoring for death or relapse) reported for patients transplanted in second complete remission is much higher than that achieved with nontransplant chemotherapy. Second, laboratory studies suggested a predictive value of 4-HC cytotoxicity on the normal hematopoietic progenitor cell for the cytotoxicity to the leukemic cells.[18] Greater 4-HC cytotoxicity resulted in lower colony-forming units–granulocyte/macrophage (CFU-GM) survival. Patients with lower CFU-GM survivals were more likely to remain in remission after transplantation. The premise of this study was that variable CFU-GM survival resulted from differing rates of inactivation of 4-HC during the incubation, and CFU-GM survival predicted the 4-HC cytotoxicity achieved against the leukemic cells. Third, similar laboratory studies from the same institution demonstrated a predictive value of the sensitivity to 4-HC of leukemic colony-forming cells (CFU-L) cultured from the marrow for the EFS of patients who underwent transplant at that center.[26] CFU-L "resistant" to 4-HC predicted for relapse. Finally, and most compelling to date, are the reports from Europe of improved EFS of selected recipients of mafosfamide-treated cells compared to similar patients who received untreated bone marrow cells (Table 8-4).[27-29] Decreased relapse rates were described for selected patients in first and second remission.

The criticism of these studies is that they may have involved highly selected patient populations. For example, increasing the

Table 8-4. Efficacy of Mafosfamide Purging for Patients Receiving Total-Body Irradiation-Containing Regimens

Patient Group	Relapse Probability	p Value	Probability of EFS	p Value
AML CR1				
Purged (N=44)	33%	0.07*	55%	0.03
Unpurged (N=102)	46%		44%	
AML CR2				
Purged (N=34)	57%	0.06	32%	0.03
Unpurged (N=30)	68%		16%	

* Shown are the significances of differences between recipients of unpurged or mafosfamide-purged bone marrow cells. (Adapted from NC Gorin, et al.[28])
EFS=event-free survival.

interval between the time at which remission is achieved and the transplant is performed decreases the probability of relapse, because patients relapsing early are excluded from the transplant group.[27] Patients referred for transplantation in second remission could, therefore, be a selected population with lower risk of relapse, and the EFS observed could reflect the treatment regimen, not the ex-vivo purge. Also, CFU-GM survival is, at best, a very indirect measure of purging efficiency. The CFU-L cultured from the marrow could represent the sensitivity of leukemic cells in the host to cyclophosphamide administered as part of the pretransplant conditioning regimen, and not the presence of clonal leukemic cells in the marrow inoculum. The European trials did not involve randomization between purging and no purging, thereby introducing the possibility of bias in those reports, and, moreover, the benefit of purging was found for only a very small subset of patients who underwent a transplant within 6 months of achieving remission and who were conditioned with total-body irradiation-containing regimens. Similar EFS has been reported after transplantation of purged or unpurged marrow to patients with AML (Table 8-5).[24,28-34]

Only limited experience in purging bone marrow cells harvested from patients with ALL has been developed in this country. The high relapse rate reported from Johns Hopkins suggests that either the conditioning regimen used or the purging technique (or both) was inadequate.[35]

Proof of efficacy of 4-HC purging for NHL, breast cancer or other maligancies is similarly lacking.

Toxicity

Treatment of bone marrow cells with activated oxazaphosphorines results in a dose-dependent loss of hematopoietic progenitors.[36-38] This may result in a delay in engraftment. Engraftment delay is most prominent for patients being treated for AML. In one series of 154 patients who received 4-HC-treated marrows, patients with AML reached $\geq$500 granulocytes/μL and platelet transfusion independence at medians of 40 and 70 days, respectively.[39] In comparison, patients being treated for intermediate or high-grade NHL reached these parameters at 20 and 30 days. Diagnosis predicted hematologic recovery independent of marrow CFU-GM content. Other significant factors were cytomegalovirus infection before either marrow harvesting or hematologic

Table 8-5. Phase II Trials of Autologous BMT in First Remission of AML

Center	Number of Patients	Time to Engraftment		Probability of		Reference
		Granulocytes	Platelets	Relapse	EFS	
A. Oxazaphosphorine-Purged Cells						
ECGBMT*	44	NS	NS	33%	NS	28
ECOG	35	31	47	11/33	54%	30
Heidelberg	22	30	71	36%	61%	25
UCSF	32	32	52	22%	76%	29
Stanford	20	31	73	28%	57%	31
B. Unpurged Cells						
ECGBMT	102	NS	NS	56%	NS	28
London	82	22	34 (to 50K)	48%	48%	33
MD Anderson	18	31	22	8/18	56%	32
FHCRC	13	29	44	67%	22%	34

* The ECGBMT and Heidelberg centers used mafosfamide for purging. Probabilities of relapse and EFS were all estimated at 2 years or more after autologous transplantation. The ECGBMT, Heidelberg, UCSF and Stanford data were extracted from reports of patients transplanted in first or later remissions or in early relapse. Granulocyte engraftment is time to achieve a peripheral blood count of ≥500µ/L; platelet engraftment is time to platelet transfusion independence. EFS=event free survival, NS=not stated, ECGBMT=European Cooperative Group for Bone Marrow Transplantation, ECOG=Eastern Cooperative Oncology Group, Heidelberg=Heidelberg University, UCSF=University of California, San Francisco, Stanford=Stanford University Medical Center, London=University College Hospital (London), MD Anderson= MD Anderson Tumor Institute, FHCRC=Fred Hutchinson Research Center.

recovery and age, with older patients engrafting faster. Experience with mafosfamide showed a similar difference in engraftment speed for patients with ALL compared to AML.[40] Gorin et al reported a significantly higher incidence of infections in recipients of mafosfamide-purged as compared to recipients of unpurged cells, as well as increased risks of hepatic venocclussive disease and interstitial pneumonitis in the nonrandomized trial in Europe.[27] However, review of 445 patients treated for a variety of malignancies at Johns Hopkins found no significant difference in infectious deaths for patients engrafting within 50 days compared to those with slower engraftment.[41] In the series from Johns Hopkins, untreated reserve cells were transfused to five of the 445 patients; those investigators could find no benefit of these reserve cells in any of these patients.[41] Three patients in this series lost marrow grafts in association with viral infection after initial hematologic recovery. Oxazaphosphorine purging may also decrease the viability of lymphocytes in the marrow inoculum.[42,43]

Recombinant growth factors may or may not hasten hematologic engraftment. Granulocyte/macrophage colony-stimulating factor (GM-CSF) did not influence engraftment of marrow that was essentially devoid of hematopoietic progenitors after 4-HC purging.[44,45] However, hematopoietic growth factors may influence the rate of engraftment for patients with malignancies other than acute leukemia despite purging with 4-HC.[46,47] This probably reflects the relationship between diagnosis and 4-HC cytotoxicity observed clinically.

Cyclophosphamide is both teratogenic and carcinogenic.[48,49] Some investigators suggested that incubation of marrow cells with activated oxazaphosphorines could induce chromosomal damage.[50] This has not been confirmed in other studies. Shah et al performed cytogenetic analysis on 55 patients after transplantation of 4-HC-treated marrow cells and found chromosomal abnormalities in 14.[51] Seven of these patients had clonal abnormalities, and all were in leukemic relapse at the time of or shortly after detection. These authors were unable to detect clonal chromosomal abnormalities that were not associated with the presence of leukemic cells after transplantation.

Purging With Other Pharmacologics

Other pharmacologic agents, including vincristine, methylprednisolone and etoposide, have been used in clinical autologous

BMT studies. In general, these agents have been used in combination with 4-HC. Two unique compounds, ether lipids and photoactive dyes, that affect the integrity of the cell membrane have been studied in Phase I or II studies.

Ether Lipids

Ether lipids produce cytotoxicity by damage to the cell membrane. This effect is relatively selective for malignant cells, possibly because of the ability of normal cells to cleave the compounds. Preclinical studies documented the ability of ex-vivo treatment to purge WEHI-3B cells from murine marrow while allowing marrow engraftment.[52] A Phase I clinical trial documented granulocyte engraftment for 23 of 24 patients receiving marrow cells treated with 50 or 75 µg/mL of edelfosine.[53] Median time to achieve ≥500 granulocytes/µL was 26 and 37 days at these two levels, respectively. One patient who received a marrow treated with 100 µg/mL failed to engraft. In-vitro cultures of hematopoietic progenitor cells showed no decrease in CFU-GM content after the marrow treatment. Ether lipid-mediated cytotoxicity is temperature-dependent and may be enhanced with incubation at hyperthermic temperatures.[54]

Photoactive Dyes

Phototoxic lipophilic drugs will bind to the cell membrane of a variety of cell types. High-affinity binding sites are found on electrically excitable cells such as neurons, immature blood cells and certain malignant cells. In the presence of plasma proteins, a differential binding to leukemic cells is achieved. On exposure of the cells to light of the correct wavelength and intensity, the cytoplasmic membrane is disrupted, and the leukemic cells swell and become trypan blue positive. The rate of photolysis depends upon dye and serum protein concentrations, and light wavelength, intensity and exposure duration.

In preclinical testing of merocyanine 540 photolysis using either broad-spectrum or argon-laser irradiation, tumor-derived cell line kills exceeding four orders of magnitude (>99.99%) were achieved while sparing 55% of multipotent hematopoietic progenitors (CFU-GEMM).[55] Merocyanine 540 photolysis did not interfere with engraftment in a murine model but was capable of preventing leukemic death after the injection into irradiated mice of 5×10^6 cells containing 1% L1210 leukemic cells.

Merocyanine 540 purging was studied in a Phase I trial at the Medical College of Wisconsin and Johns Hopkins University.[56] Twenty-one patients received marrow treated ex-vivo with merocyanine 540 and white light at one of three treatment levels. Toxic reactions to any residual dye transfused with the treated marrow were not observed. Early relapse or transplant-related morbidity precluded analysis of engraftment for nine patients. Hematologic recovery was slow, requiring 23 to 67 days to achieve 500 granulocytes/µL; three patients received transfusions of untreated "reserve" marrow because of engraftment delay beyond 6 weeks.

Combinations of Agents

Two or more pharmaceutical agents may be combined to increase the cytotoxicity against the malignant cell or decrease the cytotoxicity against the normal hematopoietic progenitor cells, or both. Combinations of drugs or drugs plus immunologic agents have been developed. Clinical experience with combinations is limited.

Chang et al demonstrated that the addition of etoposide to 4-HC was not only synergistic in cytotoxicity against a promyelocytic leukemic cell line, but was antagonistic (protective) against normal myeloid progenitor cells.[57] This effect was found at higher drug concentrations, was optimal at certain drug ratios and was found also in combination with mafosfamide.[58] Vincristine similarly may protect normal hematopoietic cells against 4-HC cytotoxicity.[59] Other drugs tested in combination with 4-HC were methylprednisolone and cisplatinum.[7,60]

Clinical experience with combination drug purging is limited. Rowley et al reported a Phase I study of purging with a combination 4-HC and vincristine followed after thorough washing by methylprednisolone (the simultaneous combination of 4-HC and methylprednisolone is toxic to normal hematopoietic progenitors).[61] They achieved a level of 4-HC in this dose-escalation study that was the same used in that laboratory for density-gradient-treated cells treated with 4-HC alone.[9] In-vitro assays for CFU-GM and CFU-L demonstrated similar survivals for the normal cells, but markedly enhanced cytotoxicity against the malignant cells from the combination drug regimen. Gulati et al reported 30 patients who received marrow cells treated with the combination of 4-HC and escalating doses of etoposide for 60 minutes at 37 C.[62] All patients engrafted at a median time to ≥500 granulocytes/μL of 32 days.

It has recently been reported that incubation of cells with amifostine (WR2721) protects the normal cells against 4-HC cytotoxicity. In a clinical study of patients being treated for breast cancer who received density-gradient-separated bone marrow cells treated with 80 μg/mL of 4-HC, those patients who received cells pretreated with amifostine reached ≥500 granulocytes/μL at a mean of 26 days, compared to 37 days for the control group (p= 0.02).[63] The experimental group also required significantly fewer platelet transfusions and days of antibiotic administration. A similar effect was seen for patients who received transplants for Hodgkin's disease or NHL.[64] The mechanism of this protection is not known. Incubation with amifostine may allow purging with higher doses of activated oxazaphosphorines, but whether this agent also protects the malignant cell has not been determined in clinical studies.

Immunologic and pharmacologic agents generally achieve cytotoxicity through different mechanisms. Combining these agents may reduce the possibility of cross-resistance to either agent, but the differing mechanisms of action are also unlikely to generate synergy. One exception may be the combination of etoposide with antibodies directed against the cell surface proteins responsible for resistance to that drug.[65]

A number of preclinical investigations have been published. In general, additive effects were found with combinations of 4-HC and immunologic agents.[66-68] Order of incubation appeared important in some studies. Investigators in Minnesota combined 4-HC with either immunotoxins or antibody and complement in the treatment of patients with lymphoid malignancies.[69,70] In the study of T-lineage ALL purged with 4-HC and immunotoxins, 82.6% to >99.96% of leukemic cells (measured by in-vitro clonogenic assays) were removed.[69] Granulocyte engraftment occurred at a median of 27 days. The second study combining 4-HC with monoclonal antibody and complement treatment for marrow samples from 14 patients reported high efficiency of malignant progenitor cell depletion in 6 patients, but relatively little depletion in 2.[69]

In neither study were the relative contributions of pharmacologic and immunologic techniques in tumor cell depletion reported.

Summary

Current data suggest that MRD may contribute to relapse after autologous BMT at least for patients with AML in first remission. Before purging should be routinely employed, however, it is necessary 1) to demonstrate that occult tumor cells may cause relapse for the disease being studied, 2) to develop an effective purging technique, 3) to prove that the purging technique decreases the probability of relapse after transplantation and 4) to prove that the purging technique improves the EFS by not increasing the toxicity of the transplant regimen. To date, improvements in risk of relapse or EFS from any of the available purging techniques have not been demonstrated. However, the toxicity of both immunologic and pharmacologic techniques is evident. Moreover, efficacy for one group of patients cannot be extrapolated to other groups. Published Phase II trials suggest that purging may benefit patients with AML, but until adequate randomized trials demonstrate an improvement in EFS, ex-vivo purging should not be routinely incorporated into the processing of hematopoietic stem cells intended for autologous transplantation for the treatment of AML or other malignant diseases.

References

1. Schultz FW, Martens ACM, Hagenbeek A. The contribution of residual leukemic cells in the graft to leukemia relapse after autologous bone marrow transplantation: Mathematical considerations. Leukemia 1989;3:530-4.
2. Hagenbeek A, Martens ACM. Cryopreservation of autologous marrow grafts in acute leukemia: survival of in vivo clonogenic leukemic cells and normal hemopoietic stem cells. Leukemia 1989;3:535-7.
3. Brenner MK, Rill DR, Moen RC, et al. Gene-marking to trace origin of relapse after autologous bone-marrow transplantation. Lancet 1993;341:85-6.
4. Blaauw A, Spitzer G, Dicke K, et al. Potential drugs for elimination of acute lymphatic leukemia cells from autologous bone marrow. Exp Hematol 1986;14:683-8.
5. Chang TT, Gulati S, Chou TC, et al. Comparative cytotoxicity of various drug combinations for human leukemic cells and normal hematopoietic precursors. Cancer Res 1987;47:119-22.

6. Gulati S, Atzpodien J, Langleben A, et al. Comparative regimens for the ex vivo chemopurification of B cell lymphoma-contaminated marrow. Acta Haematol 1988;80:65-70.
7. Jones RJ, Miller CB, Zehnbauer BA, et al. In vitro evaluation of combination drug purging for autologous bone marrow transplantation. Bone Marrow Transplant 1990;5:301-7.
8. Rowley SD. Pharmacologic purging of malignant cells. In: Forman SJ, Blume KG, Thomas ED, eds. Bone marrow transplantation. Cambridge, MA: Blackwell Scientific Publications, 1994:164-78.
9. Rowley SD, Davis JM, Piantadosi S, et al. Density-gradient separation of autologous bone marrow grafts before ex vivo purging with 4-hydroperoxycyclophosphamide. Bone Marrow Transplant 1990;6:321-7.
10. Sladek NE. Metabolism of oxazaphosphorines. Pharmacol Ther 1988;37:301-55.
11. Hilton J. Role of aldehyde dehydrogenase in cyclophosphamide-resistant L1210 leukemia. Cancer Res 1984;44:5156-60.
12. Hilton J. Deoxyribonucleic acid crosslinking by 4-hydroperoxycyclophosphamide in cyclophosphamide-sensitive and -resistant L1210 cells. Biochem Pharmacol 1984;33:1867-72.
13. Kohn FR, Landkamer GJ, Manthey CL, et al. Effect of aldehyde dehydrogenase inhibitors on the ex vivo sensitivity of human multipotent and committed hematopoietic progenitor cells and malignant blood cells to oxazaphosphorines. Cancer Res 1987;47:3180-5.
14. Sahovic EA, Colvin M, Hilton J, Ogawa M. Role for aldehyde dehydrogenase in survival of progenitors for murine blast cell colonies after treatment with 4-hydroperoxycyclophosphamide in vitro. Cancer Res 1988;48:1223-6.
15. Gordon MY, Goldman JM, Gordon-Smith EC. 4-Hydroperoxycyclophosphamide inhibits proliferation by human granulocyte-macrophage colony-forming cells (GM-CFC) but spares more primitive progenitor cells. Leuk Res 1985;9:1017-21.
16. Kastan MB, Schlaffer E, Russo JE, et al. Direct demonstration of elevated aldehyde dehydrogenase in human hematopoietic progenitor cells. Blood 1990;75:1947-50.
17. Jones RJ, Zuehlsdorf M, Rowley SD, et al. Variability in 4-hydroperoxycyclophosphamide activity during clinical

purging for autologous bone marrow transplantation. Blood 1987;70:1490-4.

18. Rowley SD, Jones RJ, Piantadosi S, et al. Efficacy of ex vivo purging for autologous bone marrow transplantation in the treatment of acute nonlymphoblastic leukemia. Blood 1989;74:501-6.

19. Herve P, Tamayo E, Peters A. Autologous stem cell grafting in acute myeloid leukemia: Technical approach of marrow incubation in vitro with pharmacologic agents (prerequisite for clinical applications). Br J Haematol 1983;53:683-5.

20. Sharkis S, Santos GW, Colvin M. Elimination of acute myelogenous leukemic cells from marrow and tumor suspensions in the rat with 4-hydroperoxycyclophosphamide. Blood 1980;55:521-3.

21. Yeager AM, Kaizer H, Santos GW, et al. Autologous bone marrow transplantation in patients with acute non-lymphocytic leukemia using ex vivo marrow treatment with 4-hydroperoxycyclophosphamide. N Engl J Med 1986;315:141-7.

22. Gorin NC, Douay L, Laporte JP, et al. Autologous bone marrow transplantation using marrow incubated with Asta Z 7557 in adult acute leukemia. Blood 1986;67:1367-76.

23. Rosenfeld C, Shadduck RK, Przepiorka D, et al. Autologous bone marrow transplantation with 4-hydroperoxycyclophosphamide purged marrows for acute nonlymphocytic leukemia in late remission or early relapse. Blood 1989;74:1159-64.

24. Lenarsky C, Weinberg K, Petersen J, et al. Autologous bone marrow transplantation with 4-hydroperoxycyclophosphamide purged marrows for children with acute non-lymphoblastic leukemia in second remission. Bone Marrow Transplant 1990;6:425-9.

25. Korbling M, Hunstein W, Fliedner TM, et al. Disease-free survival after autologous bone marrow transplantation in patients with acute myelogenous leukemia. Blood 1989;74:1898-904.

26. Miller CB, Zehnbauer BA, Piantadosi S, et al. Correlation of occult clonogenic leukemia drug sensitivity with relapse after autologous bone marrow transplantation. Blood 1991;78:1125-31.

27. Gorin NC, Aegerter P, Auvert B, et al. Autologous bone marrow transplantation for acute myelocytic leukemia in

first remission: A European survey of the role of marrow purging. Blood 1990;75:1606-14.

28. Gorin NC, Labopin M, Meloni G, et al. Autologous bone marrow transplantation for acute myeloblastic leukemia in Europe: Further evidence of the role of marrow purging by mafosfamide. Leukemia 1991;5:896-904.

29. Linker CA, Ries CA, Damon LE, et al. Autologous bone marrow transplantation for acute myeloid leukemia using busulfan plus etoposide as a preparative regimen. Blood 1993;81:311-8.

30. Cassileth PA, Andersen J, Lazarus HM, et al. Autologous bone marrow transplant in acute myeloid leukemia in first remission. J Clin Oncol 1993;11:314-9.

31. Chao NJ, Stein AS, Long GD, et al. Busulfan/etoposide—initial experience with a new preparatory regimen for autologous bone marrow transplantation in patients with acute nonlymphoblastic leukemia. Blood 1993;81:319-23.

32. Spinolo JA, Dicke KA, Horwitz LJ, et al. Double intensification with amsacrine/high dose ara-C and high dose chemotherapy with autologous bone marrow transplantation produces durable remissions in acute myelogenous leukemia. Bone Marrow Transplant 1990;5:111-8.

33. McMillan AK, Goldstone AH, Linch DC, et al. High-dose chemotherapy and autologous bone marrow transplantation in acute myeloid leukemia. Blood 1990;76:480-8.

34. Stewart P, Buckner CD, Bensinger W, et al. Autologous marrow transplantation in patients with acute nonlymphocytic leukemia in first remission. Exp Hematol 1985;13:267-72.

35. Santos GW, Yeager AM, Jones RJ. Autologous bone marrow transplantation. Annu Rev Med 1989,40:99-112.

36. Rowley SD, Colvin OM, Stuart RK. Human multilineage progenitor cell sensitivity to 4-hydroperoxycyclophosphamide. Exp Hematol 1985;13:295-8.

37. Siena S, Castro-Malaspina H, Gulati S, et al. Effects of in vitro purging with 4-hydroperoxycyclophosphamide on the hematopoietic and microenvironmental elements of human bone marrow. Blood 1985;65:655-62.

38. Winton EF, Colenda KW. Use of long-term human marrow cultures to demonstrate progenitor cell precursors in marrow treated with 4-hydroperoxycyclophosphamide. Exp Hematol 1987;15:710-14.

39. Rowley SD, Piantadosi S, Marcellus DC, et al. Analysis of factors predicting speed of hematologic recovery after transplantation with 4-hydroperoxycyclophosphamide-purged autologous bone marrow grafts. Bone Marrow Transplant 1991;7:183-91.

40. Douay L, Laporte JP, Mary JY, et al. Difference in kinetics of hematopoietic reconstitution between ALL and ANLL after autologous bone marrow transplantation with marrow treated in vitro with mafosfamide (ASTA Z 7557). Bone Marrow Transplant 1987;2:33-43.

41. Davis JM, Rowley SD, Piantadosi S, et al. Graft failure after 4-hydroperoxycyclophosphamide (4-HC)-purged autologous bone marrow transplantation (ABMT) (abstract). Blood 1992;80(suppl 1):376a.

42. Korbling M, Hess AD, Tutschka PJ, et al. 4-Hydroperoxycyclophosphamide: A model for eliminating residual human tumour cells and T-lymphocytes from the bone marrow graft. Br J Haematol 1982;52:89-96.

43. Le Blanc G, Douay L, Laporte JP, et al. Evaluation of lymphocyte subsets after autologous bone marrow transplantation with marrow treated by ASTA Z 7557 in acute leukemia: Incidence of the in vitro treatment. Exp Hematol 1986;14:366-71.

44. Nemunaitis J, Singer JW, Buckner CD, et al. Use of recombinant human granulocyte-macrophage colony-stimulating factor in graft failure after bone marrow transplantation. Blood 1990;76:245-53.

45. Blazar BR, Kersey JH, McGlave PB, et al. In vivo administration of recombinant human granulocyte/macrophage colony-stimulating factor in acute lymphoblastic leukemia patients receiving purged autografts. Blood 1989;73:849-57.

46. Gorin NC, Coiffier B, Hayat M, et al. Recombinant human granulocyte-macrophage colony-stimulating factor after high-dose chemotherapy and autologous bone marrow transplantation with unpurged and purged marrow in non-Hodgkin's lymphoma: A double-blind placebo-controlled trial. Blood 1992;80:1149-57.

47. Carlo-Stella C, Mangoni L, Almici C, et al. Use of recombinant human granulocyte-macrophage colony-stimulating factor in patients with lymphoid malignancies transplanted with unpurged or adjusted-dose mafosfamide-purged autologous marrow. Blood 1992;80:2412-18.

48. Friedman OM, Myles A, Colvin M. Cyclophosphamide and related phosphoramide mustards. Current status and future prospects. Adv Cancer Chemother 1979;1:143-204.
49. Perocco P, Pane G, Santucci A, Zannotti M. Mutagenic and toxic effects of 4-hydroperoxycyclophosphamide and of 2,4-tetrahydrocyclohexylamine (ASTA-Z-7557) on human lymphocytes cultured in vitro. Exp Hematol 1985;13:1014-7.
50. Van Den Akker J, Gorin NC, Laporte JP, et al. Chromosomal abnormalities after autologous bone marrow transplantation with marrow treated by cyclophosphamide derivatives. Lancet 1985;1:1211-12.
51. Shah NK, Wingard J, Piantadosi S, et al. Chromosome abnormalities in patients treated with 4-hydroperoxycyclophosphamide-purged autologous bone marrow transplantation. Cancer Genet Cytogenet 1993;65:135-40.
52. Glasser L, Somberg LB, Vogler WR. Purging murine leukemic marrow with alkyl-lysophospholipids. Blood 1984;64:1288-91.
53. Vogler WR, Berdel WE, Olson AC, et al. Autologous bone marrow transplantation in acute leukemia with marrow purged with alkyl-lysophospholipid. Blood 1992;80:1423-9.
54. Okamoto S, Olson AC, Berdel WE, Vogler WR. Purging of acute myeloid leukemic cells by ether lipids and hyperthermia. Blood 1988;72:1777-83.
55. Sieber F, Rao S, Rowley SD, Sieber-Blum M. Dye-mediated photolysis of human neuroblastoma cells: Implications for autologous bone marrow transplantation. Blood 1986;68:32-6.
56. Sieber F. Extracorporeal purging of bone marrow grafts by dye-sensitized photoirradiation. In: Gee AP, ed. Bone marrow processing and purging. A practical guide. Boca Raton: CRC Press, 1991:263-80.
57. Chang TT, Gulati SC, Chou TC, et al. Synergistic effect of 4-hydroperoxycyclophosphamide and etoposide on a human promyelocyte leukemia cell line (HL-60) demonstrated by computer analysis. Cancer Res 1985;45:2434-9.
58. De Faritiis P, Pulsoni A, Sandrelli A, et al. Efficacy of a combined treatment with ASTA-Z 7654 and VP16-213 in vitro in eradicating clonogenic tumor cells from human bone marrow. Bone Marrow Transplant 1987;2:287-98.

59. Auber ML, Horwitz LJ, Blaauw A, et al. Evaluation of drugs for elimination of leukemic cells from the bone marrow of patients with acute leukemia. Blood 1988;71:166-72.
60. Peters RH, Brandon CS, Avila LA, et al. In vitro synergism of 4-hydroperoxycyclophosphamide and cisplatin: relevance for bone marrow purging. Cancer Chemother Pharmacol 1989;23:129-34.
61. Rowley SD, Miller CD, Piantadosi S, et al. Phase I study of combination drug purging for autologous bone marrow transplantation. J Clin Oncol 1991;9:2210-8.
62. Gulati SC, Acaba L, Yahalom J, et al. Autologous bone marrow transplantation for acute myelogenous leukemia using 4-hydroperoxycyclophosphamide and VP-16 purged bone marrow. Bone Marrow Transplant 1992;10:129-34.
63. Shpall EJ, Jones RB, Johnston C, et al. Amifostine (WR-2721) shortens the engraftment period of 4-HC purged bone marrow in breast cancer patients receiving high-dose chemotherapy with autologous bone marrow support (ABMS) (abstract). Blood 1991;78(suppl 1):192a.
64. Stemmer SM, Shpall EJ, Jones RB, et al. Amifostine (WR-2721) shortens the engraftment time of 4-hydroperoxycyclophosphamide (4-HC) purged bone marrow in lymphoma patients receiving high-dose chemotherapy (HDC) with autologous bone marrow support (ABMS) (abstract). Blood 1992;80(suppl 1):70a.
65. Aihara M, Aihara Y, Schmidt-Wolf G, et al. A combined approach for purging multidrug-resistant leukemic cell lines in bone marrow using a monoclonal antibody and chemotherapy. Blood 1991;77:2079-84.
66. De Fabritiis P, Bregni M, Lipton J, et al. Elimination of clonogenic Burkitt's lymphoma cells from human bone marrow using 4-hydroperoxycyclophosphamide in combination with monoclonal antibodies and complement. Blood 1985;65:1064-70.
67. Lemoli RM, Gasparetto C, Scheinberg DA, et al. Autologous bone marrow transplantation in acute myelogenous leukemia: In vitro treatment with myeloid-specific monoclonal antibodies and drugs in combination. Blood 1991;77:1829-36.
68. Uckun FM, Gajl-Peczalska K, Meyers DE, et al. Marrow purging in autologous bone marrow transplantation for T-lineage acute lymphoblastic leukemia: Efficacy of ex vivo

treatment with immunotoxins and 4-hydroperoxycyclophosphamide against fresh leukemic marrow progenitor cells. Blood 1987;69:361-6.

69. Uckun FM, Kersey JH, Vallera DA, et al. Autologous bone marrow transplantation in high risk remission T-lineage acute lymphoblastic leukemia using immunotoxins plus 4-hydroperoxycyclophosphamide for marrow purging. Blood 1990;76:1723-33.

70. Uckun FM, Kersey JH, Haake R, et al. Autologous bone marrow transplantation in high-risk remission B-lineage acute lymphoblastic leukemia using a cocktail of three monoclonal antibodies (BA-1/CD24, BA-2/CD9, and BA-3/CD10) plus complement and 4-hydroperoxycyclophosphamide for ex vivo bone marrow purging. Blood 1992;79:1094-104.

In: Lasky L and Warkentin P, eds. *Marrow and Stem Cell Processing for Transplantation*
Bethesda, MD: American Association of Blood Banks, 1995

9

T-Cell Depletion of Allogeneic Bone Marrow Transplants by Immunologic and Physical Techniques

Nancy H. Collins, PhD; Adrian P. Gee, PhD; and P. Jean Henslee-Downey, MD

THE USE OF HLA-MATCHED or partially matched allogeneic bone marrow from normal donors, usually family members, in the treatment of hematologic malignancies, bone marrow failure or immunodeficiency syndromes offers certain advantages to the recipient. Normal allogeneic marrow is often the preferred option in malignancies in which neoplastic cells infiltrate the autologous marrow. In addition, the normal marrow from an allogeneic donor may confer immunologic control of the residual neoplastic cells remaining after conditioning of the recipient, the graft-vs-leukemic (GVL) effect. In bone marrow failure states, eg, aplastic anemia or congenital immunodeficiency diseases, in which autologous recovery of normal hematopoiesis is not an option, the only source of hematologically normal cells is an allogeneic donor.[1]

Nancy H. Collins, PhD, Laboratory Director, Allogeneic Bone Marrow Processing, Charles A. Dana Bone Marrow Transplant Unit, Memorial Sloan-Kettering Cancer Center, New York, New York; Adrian P. Gee, PhD, Professor of Medicine and Director for Applied Research, Division of Transplantation Medicine, Center for Cancer Treatment and Research, Richland Memorial Hospital, University of South Carolina, Columbia, South Carolina; and P. Jean Henslee-Downey, MD, Professor of Medicine and Pediatrics and Director, Division of Transplantation Medicine, Center for Cancer Treatment and Research, Richland Memorial Hospital, University of South Carolina, Columbia, South Carolina
[This work has been supported by grant CA23766 from the National Cancer Institute (NHC) and a research gift from Baxter Biotech - Immunotherapy (APG).]

Histocompatibility

The biggest obstacle to the use of allogeneic bone marrow transplantation (BMT) is the histocompatiblity system—both major and minor antigens. Increasingly sophisticated methods to define histocompatiblity antigens have contributed materially to the success of BMT. The elucidation of the molecular structure of the major histocompatibility complex (MHC) antigens and the genetic material underlying their expression has greatly expanded the techniques that can be used to match BMT donors and recipients. The classic methods of serologic typing for Class I antigens and mixed lymphocyte culture reactivities for Class II antigens have been supplemented by newer technologies. Class I antigens can be analyzed by isoelectric focusing of radiolabeled immunoprecipitates. Class II antigens can be compared by using the DNA-based analyses of restriction length polymorphisms and sequence-specific or allele-specific oligonucleotide probes.[2,3]

Other measures of lymphocyte responses that can be used in donor-recipient pairs are the CTL_p and HTL_p assays, which employ limiting-dilution analysis of lymphocytes responding to allogeneic antigens giving rise to a cytotoxic reactivity or interleukin-2 (IL-2) production.[4,5]

Graft-vs-Host Disease

Etiology

The primary complication associated with the transplantation of allogeneic bone marrow for malignancies and bone marrow failure is graft-vs-host disease (GVHD).[6] This results from the recognition of unshared allogeneic histocompatibility antigens on the recipient's cells by immunocompetent T cells in the graft. The reaction occurs in up to 80% of HLA-matched sibling transplants, which indicates that it may be mediated by minor histocompatibility differences not detected by conventional HLA-matching techniques. The role of T cells in initiating the reaction was first shown in animal experiments[7] and confirmed in humans by the demonstration that ex-vivo depletion of T cells from the graft abrogated or reduced the incidence and severity of GVHD in the recipients.[8] Since a similar reaction has been reported in syngeneic and autologous transplants, where there is no antigenic difference between donor and recipient, it is clear that

GVHD may arise by a number of mechanisms, including an imbalance in immunity in the posttransplant period.[9]

Both CD4+ and CD8+ donor T cells have been implicated in the initiation of GVHD, which is then amplified by the production of IL-2 by T-helper cells. The primary targets for these cells are the proliferating cells in the recipient's gastrointestinal tract and epithelium, where attack is directed toward the basal layers of the skin and the intestinal submucosa. Pancytopenia and immune suppression may also be produced as a result of effects upon the bone marrow and lymphoid system. Common features shared by these target cells are the expression of Class II antigens and the fact that the cells are in cycle.

Clinical Symptoms

Acute GVHD is usually initially manifested as a rash over the face, neck, ears, soles, palms and extensor surface of the limbs. The rash may spread and become confluent with the development of fever, erythema, blistering and eventual desquamation.[6] Definitive diagnosis by skin biopsy may be difficult, since the initial symptoms may resemble those produced by chemoradiotherapy.

Involvement of the gastrointestinal tract and liver usually occurs after the skin reaction. Typically, diarrhea and nausea develop accompanied by abdominal cramps and loss of appetite. Cholestatic jaundice is common.

If symptoms are still evident at 100 days after BMT, the reaction is usually reclassified as chronic GVHD, although the acute and chronic forms may occur independently and in isolation. Chronic GVHD is characterized by sclerosis and atrophy of the dermis and is graded I through IV by the number and severity of involvement of organs and systems. Symptoms include skin lesions, cytopenia, lymphoid atrophy, recurrent infections, liver dysfunction, ulceration of gut mucosa and autoantibody formation. Ultimately, GVHD is associated directly or indirectly with 25% of the mortality seen after BMT.

Both in-vivo and ex-vivo depletion of T cells may be used to prevent GVHD. This chapter discusses ex-vivo removal of T cells and T-cell subsets. In-vivo methods to block T cells include administration of cyclosporine, infusion of T-cell-directed monoclonal antibodies (MoAbs) and the use of antibodies directed against the IL-2 receptor. Cytotoxic agents such as methotrexate and cyclophosphamide may be useful in preventing mild GVHD but are not effective for preventing the severe and lethal forms of the reaction. Steroid treatment is effective for prevention only when used in combination with other agents. Cyclosporin A has shown the most promise for GVHD prevention and probably acts at both the recognition and amplification phases of the disease. Therapeutic serum levels should be achieved prior to BMT and maintained for up to one year after transplant.[6,9]

Treatment of acute GVHD usually involves steroid administration. Disease that is refractory to this therapy has a poor prognosis, with progression to chronic GVHD and up to 80% mortality. Chronic GVHD is also treated with steroids in combination with a variety of other agents, including antithymocyte globulin, cyclosporine, azathioprine, thalidomide and lymph node irradiation.

In conclusion, GVHD is one of the most serious complications of allogeneic BMT occurring to various degrees in the majority of recipients and accounting directly or indirectly for up to 25% of deaths. The most effective method for preventing this reaction is the depletion of T cells from the donor marrow before transplantation; however, the use of this procedure is associated with a number of additional complications.[6,9]

The Paradox of T-Cell Depletion in Allogeneic Transplantation

It has been well demonstrated in animal model systems that the inactivation or physical removal of donor T cells eliminates the potentially lethal sequelae of GVHD in allogeneic BMT.[10] T-cell depletion (TCD) was introduced into the clinic in the 1970s with encouraging results. The initial enthusiasm for TCD resulted in the application of a wide variety of methods of bone marrow treatment to more than 800 transplants between 1981 and 1986. Indeed, the reduction or elimination of GVHD allowed the extension of this therapeutic option to patients who lack an HLA-compatible donor and to older transplant recipients for whom GVHD is a more serious complication than it is for children. TCD further reduced the need for and complications of posttransplant GVHD prophylaxis.[11]

The results of TCD varied from center to center, by patient population, disease state and remission status. However, the gains in survival of the recipients of TCD grafts that are attributable to the diminution of GVHD and its attendant infectious complications were offset by increased risks of graft failure/rejection. Increased leukemic relapse rates after transplant were seen in some diseases.[12,13] Other problems included the appearance of donor-type lymphoproliferative disease posttransplant. Further, while the kinetics of engraftment were similar for unmodified and TCD transplants, there was evidence of differences in the immunologic reconstitution in the two groups. While the analysis of immune reconstitution is complicated by the immunosuppressive effects of GVHD and GVHD prophylaxis, it can be inferred that alteration of the cell types contained in a hematopoietic graft can have profound effects on the recovery of immune function.[14]

Renewed interest in TCD has, however, been spurred by the use of unrelated HLA-matched donors for patients lacking a matched related donor.[15] New technologies in cell selection that can be adapted to T-cell selection, both negative and positive, increase the ease of manipulating and standardizing bone marrow treatment. T-cell-depleted BMT also became a more attractive model for the study of T-cell function following more sophisticated definition of T-cell subpopulations. Finally, newer methods of patient support using cytokines posttransplant offer insight into the interactive network of factors affecting engraftment. [16]

Evaluation of T-Cell-Depleted Bone Marrow

T-cell depletion alters bone marrow in a measurable fashion, which poses special challenges for the evaluation of the treated marrow. Manipulation of bone marrow often results not only in the concentration of the hematopoietic precursors, as T cells are removed or inactivated, but also in the loss of cells other than the targeted T cells. Careful monitoring of percent of recovery of total cell numbers, identification of remaining cell populations and recovery of clonable hematopoietic precursors and residual T cells at various stages of TCD are required for analysis of the success of the depletion and correlation with clinical outcome.

T cells are well-defined phenotypically, functionally and by molecular techniques. Assays for residual T cells vary in their sensitivity and utility in the evaluation of T-cell-depleted marrow. Further, the method of TCD used determines the proper assay to measure residual T cells. The more complete or successful the depletion, the more difficult is the detection of residual T cells. It has been established in several systems, that more than 99% of T cells must be removed from a standard bone marrow harvest in order to reduce the level of GVHD to acceptable levels.[17]

Several standard laboratory measures of T-cell content are of limited utility in T-cell-depleted marrow. Analytical rosetting that measures the CD2+ T and natural killer cells, while a quick and standard laboratory technique, is of limited sensitivity and is dependent on the number of cells examined. Furthermore, rosettes are susceptible to mechanical disruption. Bulk proliferative responses to T cell mitogens or allogeneic cells in T-cell-depleted marrow are hampered by the high rate of background proliferation in bone marrow.[18]

Flow cytometry presently is a powerful tool in the analysis of T-cell-depleted marrow that can be applied before the graft is administered. Clinical TCD expanded during the era of phenomenal development in flow cytometry and the definition of multiple, easily detectable antigenic markers for T cells. The development of directly fluoresceinated CD34 antibodies has simplified the examination of bone marrow. While CD34+ cells occur in low frequencies in normal marrow, they are often concentrated and thus easier to detect in T-cell-depleted marrow. Both CD34+ hematopoietic progenitor cells and T cells are easily gated in the lymphoblastoid area defined by forward and orthogonal light scatter in a standard cytogram. The ability to gate these cells together both eliminates the high autoflurorescence of the larger and more granular myeloid cells and increases the percentage of the rare CD34+ cell before depletion and the rare T cell after depletion (Fig 9-1). Yet, the sensitivity of flow cytometric analysis in most laboratories is approximately 1%, which falls well above the limit of T-cell content for the prediction of GVHD.

Table 9-1 presents the phenotypic analysis of bone marrow after TCD by soybean lectin agglutinin (SBA) agglutination and adherence on covalently immobilized CD5 and CD8 MoAbs. The number of cells in the lymphoblastoid gate decreases with increasing TCD. Examination of the lymphoblastoid gate shows the decrease in T-cell markers coupled with the increase in CD34+ cells more clearly than does the calculation of the percent of recovery for the entire population.[19]

The first measure of residual T cells shown to correlate with GVHD in HLA-matched T-cell-depleted grafts was the T-cell outgrowth assay by limiting-dilution analysis in the presence of IL-2-containing medium from the gibbon cell line MLA and the mitogen PHA 16.[20] This very sensitive assay, in which the frequency

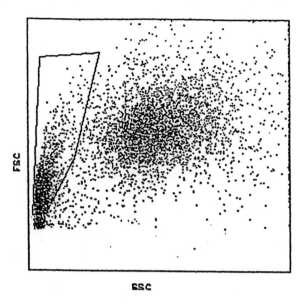

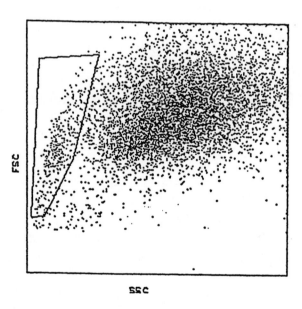

Figure 9-1. Cytogram of the forward vs orthogonal scatter of RBC-depleted bone marrow (top) and bone marrow depleted of T cells by agglutination with SBA and passage over the AIS CD5/CD8 CELL-ector-T cell (bottom). The gate was set on the lymphoblastoid population, determined by presence of T lymphocyte markers and the CD34+CD33– populations and the absence of myeloid markers.

Table 9-1. Expression of Phenotypic Markers During Successive Steps of T-Cell Depletion by SBA Agglutination and Adherence on the CD5/CD8 Cellector

Antigen	Unseparated	SBA-*	SBA- (CD5/CD8)-*
CD2	40.0 (8.9)	75.5 (14.4)	29.7 (2.0)
CD4	21.6 (4.8)	19.1 (3.6)	15.7 (1.0)
CD5	48.9 (10.9)	70.9 (13.5)	9.2 (0.6)
CD8	24.0 (5.4)	38.9 (7.4)	4.0 (0.3)
CD34	0.7 (0.2)	2.8 (0.5)	11.3 (0.7)
CD56	5.5 (1.2)	9.8 (1.8)	4.7 (0.3)
% cells in gate	22.3	19.1	6.7

* % gated (% entire cell population)

of clonable T cells is determined by microscopic evaluation, uses small numbers of cells, but requires 12 days of incubation. The $\log_{10}$ depletion of the method under analysis is the $\log_{10}$ of the quotient of the total number of clonable T cells in the harvested marrow divided by the total number of T cells in the T-cell-depleted marrow. While the total number of T cells varies from harvest to harvest, a $\log_{10}$ of 1.5 - 3.0 is usually sufficient to reduce the number of clonable T cells to below the 1×10^5/kg dose that has been defined as predictive of a 50% chance of Grade I GVHD in HLA-matched T-cell-depleted transplants for leukemia. [21]

Assays for hematopoietic progenitors are routinely used on bone marrow both before and after TCD. The techniques commonly in use measure committed hematopoietic progenitor cells, resulting in conflicting reports as to their correlation with clinical engraftment. Techniques defining more primitive hematopoietic progenitors have been developed and applied to various TCD methods. [22] It is generally recognized that standardization is sorely needed in this area. Calculation of total recovery of progenitors from T-cell-depleted bone marrow is more difficult to evaluate by any one of the culture systems, because of the effect of altered interactions between cell populations before and after TCD, which results in gain or loss of suppressive or stimulatory activity. Recoveries in excess of 100% of any one clonogenic precursor type are not unusual.

Table 9-2 shows a comparison between bone marrow harvests that have undergone TCD by two different methods (see lectin-

Table 9-2. Comparison of SBA– Cells Depleted of T Cells by Treatment With the AIS CD5/CD8 Cellector-T Cell or by Rosetting With Sheep RBCs

	SBA–(5/8)– Grafts (Mean ± SD)	SBA–E– Grafts (Mean ± SD)	P Value
A. Cell Recovery			
Harvested marrow			
Total × 10^9	27.9 ± 5.8	25.9 ± 7.8	0.302
RBC depleted			
Total × 10^9	18.3 ± 5.0	15.6 ± 5.0	0.058
SBA–			
Total × 10^9	3.2 ± 1.3	3.2 ± 1.7	0.970
%RBC Depleted	17.3 ± 4.9	21.0 ± 6.7	0.028
T-cell depleted			
Total × 10^9	2.6 ± 1.1	1.7 ± 0.8	0.001
%SBA–	81.7 ± 9.4	54.8 ± 13.9	<0.001
B. T-Cell Number			
RBC Depleted			
% E+	16.3 ± 5.5	13.8 ± 5.2	0.096
Total # E+ (× 10^9)	2.9 ± 1.0	2.0 ± 0.8	0.002
SBA–			
% E+	11.3 ± 6.0	9.0 ± 4.0	0.107
Total # E+ (× 10^8)	3.4 ± 2.1	3.0 ± 2.0	0.449
T-Cell Depleted			
% E+	1.0 ± 0.9	0.0 ± 0.1	<0.001
Clonable T cells (× 10^6)	2.3 ± 1.6	1.2 ± 1.2	0.065
Log$_{10}$ TCD by LDA	2.4 ± 0.3	2.6 ± 0.3	0.140
C. CFU-GM			
RBC Depleted			
Total × 10^6	10.2 ± 4.0	8.6 ± 5.4	0.258
T-Cell Depleted			
Total × 10^6	4.3 ± 2.2	4.5 ± 2.8	0.809
%RBC Depleted	45.9 ± 29.7	53.8 ± 23.7	0.305
D. BFU-E			
RBC Depleted			
Total × 10^6	8.2 ± 7.1	4.9 ± 4.0	0.044
T-Cell Depleted			
Total × 10^6	2.2 ± 1.3	2.3 ± 1.4	0.951
%RBC Depleted	45.4 ± 26.4	51.1 ± 26.4	0.566

based techniques below). The bone marrow samples were compared at successive stages of depletion by assays of total cell numbers, numbers of T cells determined by rosetting and limiting-dilution T-cell outgrowth assays, and numbers of clonogenic hematopoietic progenitor cells. Substantial differences are seen in percent of recovery of total cell numbers, while recovery of T-cell numbers in the final product is similar in the two groups. Thus, the final $\log_{10}$ TCD is not significantly different. The total recovery of hematopoietic progenitor cells shows an extremely large standard deviation, reflecting broad variation in recovery among marrow samples, whichever method is used for TCD.[23]

T-Cell Depletion Methods

In a recent worldwide survey of bone marrow processing laboratories, it was reported that TCD of some type was used by 28% of North American laboratories, 46% of European laboratories and 17% of laboratories in other parts of the world. MoAb-based techniques were used in 22%, 57% and 50% of the laboratories, respectively. Immunotoxin techniques, in which the MoAb of interest is conjugated to a toxin that then kills the T cell after binding, accounted for the TCD in 14% of North American laboratories and in 4% of European laboratories. Physical removal of T cells was accomplished in these laboratories by counterflow centrifugation elutriation (CCE) in 18%, 26% and 0% of the reporting laboratories, respectively. The remainder of the reporting centers utilized a lectin-based technique in which the first step of TCD was concentration of hematopoietic precursors with a 1 $\log_{10}$ depletion of T cells by agglutination with or binding to SBA (29% of North American and 37% of European centers).[24]

Immunophysical Techniques for T-Cell Depletion

Immunophysical techniques for the depletion of T cells from allogeneic grafts use MoAbs to identify and mediate the separation of the target cells from the marrow. Depending upon the particular application, either pan-T (eg, anti-CD3, CD2, CD5, etc) or T-cell-subset-directed antibodies (eg, anti-CD8) are used. In most cases, the antibodies are immobilized on a solid phase matrix that is then incubated with the marrow. Separation of the

T cells is achieved by removal of the solid phase from the cell suspension. Suitable matrices include polystyrene plates, Sepharose™ particles and paramagnetic microspheres, particles or colloids. These approaches have been used extensively for purging tumor cells from marrow that is to be used for autologous transplantation and are discussed in detail in Chapter 6. In the case of TCD, a number of points should be made.

In general, T lymphocytes and T-cell subsets display a more homogeneous expression of antigens than do tumor cells. This facilitates separation using a single MoAb, whereas it is normal to use panels of antibodies for tumor depletion to compensate for the heterogeneous expression of any single antigen. In addition, satisfactory results may often be obtained by coupling the antibody to the solid phase, eg, a magnetic bead, rather than by adding the MoAb to the marrow and then incubating it with a solid phase coated with immunoglobulin antibody—the indirect technique. This results in a considerable saving of time and reduces manipulation of the cells.

In tumor cell depletion, it is normal to set an upper limit for infiltration of the marrow by tumor cells. Above that limit, purging will not be performed or may not produce satisfactory results. In T-cell purging, the concentration of potential target cells within the harvested marrow may vary considerably, due to the admixture of the cells with peripheral blood during the harvest. Any method that is developed must be capable of achieving the desired level of depletion, starting with the maximum anticipated T-cell burden in the graft. If the aim is to return a specific number and subtype of T cells to the patient, then the method must also be capable of adaptation to achieve this end when starting with very heterogeneous initial cell populations. Immunophysical separation methods offer particular promise in this area since the target cells may be recovered from the solid phase and, if necessary, be added back to the graft.

This inherent variability in the size of the potential target cell population within the graft may in turn affect the applicability of different approaches to cell separation. Although immunomagnetic separation has been shown to be effective for TCD on a small scale, when scaled up to treat a clinically appropriate volume of material containing a high percentage of T cells, it may become costly and require modification to ensure efficient capture of the cells within the magnetic field. Alternatively, the cells may have to be processed in smaller batches, adding to both the variability and length of the procedure. In the case of conventional panning, the larger target cell burden may require extremely large surface areas to immobilize sufficient antibody to achieve satisfactory levels of TCD. This may make the separation device physically cumbersome. In both approaches, a solution is to perform an initial bulk depletion of T cells, eg, by using elutriation or SBA, and then to "fine tune" the separation using immunophysical approaches.

The development of TCD methods is somewhat simpler than is the case with tumor purging systems. Peripheral blood can be used in model experiments to optimize separation conditions and marrow can be substituted in later tests to confirm the results. Assays for validating the performance of the systems are readily available in the form of both limiting-dilution analysis and multidimensional flow cytometry. In both cases, the same assays can then be used to monitor the clinical performance of the technique.

An alternative approach to immunophysical separation is the use of MoAbs to target agents that are toxic to the T cells. For example, antibody-sensitized cells may be destroyed by the addition of serum complement, either supplied by the recipient of the graft as autologous serum or added exogenously as baby rabbit serum. Although the use of complement is associated with a number of problems, successful studies using this technique have been reported.[25] Depletion of 1.5-2.5 $\log_{10}$ of T cells (Fig 9-2) bearing the T-cell receptor $\alpha\beta$ heterodimer from partially matched, related allografts, using the T10B9 MoAb and rabbit complement, facilitated mismatched transplants with good engraftment of the treated marrow and manageable GVHD. Alternatively, a toxin, such as ricin from the castor bean or diphtheria toxin, may be directly conjugated to the MoAb and once incorporated into the T cell, it will mediate its destruction.[26] This method, primarily using anti-CD5 or anti-CD3 conjugates, is capable of achieving high levels of TCD (>3 $\log_{10}$), but this resulted in graft failure in early studies. T-cell subset depletion using anti-CD8 immunotoxins may resolve this problem while exploiting the specificity and potency of immunotoxin-based depletion.

Physical Depletion of T Cells

Counterflow Centrifugation Elutriation

CCE takes advantage of the differences in cell size and density of T lymphocytes and other marrow components. This technique

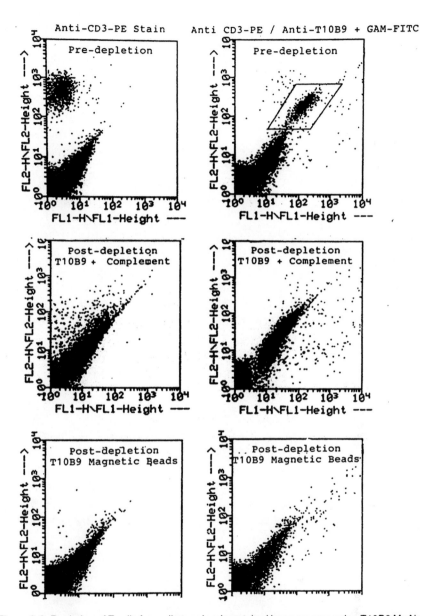

Figure 9-2. Depletion of T cells from allogeneic mismatched bone marrow using T10B9 MoAb. Depletion was analyzed using flow cytometric analysis and staining with anti-CD3 MoAb conjugated to phycoerythrin (left column, ordinate) or dual screening (right column) with anti-CD3-PE (ordinate) and anti-T10B9 plus fluorescein isothiocyanate (FITC)-conjugated goat anti-mouse (GAM) immunoglogulin (abscissa). Target T cells are shown in the box in the upper right panel. Top two panels are predepletion values. The center panels show residual T cells following clinical scale depletion using T10B9 and complement. The lower panels show residual T cells following small-scale depletion using T10B9 adsorbed to paramagnetic microspheres. A 2.7 $\log_{10}$ depletion was obtained by T10B9 plus complement as determined by limiting-dilution analysis.

subjects a buffy coat from a normal marrow to simultaneous opposing forces from centrifugation and medium flow. Cell fractions are collected at various flow rates of medium or in the stationary (rotor off) position. The major advantage of CCE is that all cells can be recovered from the various fractions without alteration in their function, so that combinations may be made of well-characterized cell populations. In this way, the patient can receive a graft with a predetermined dose of lymphocytes. The hematopoietic progenitor-rich fraction is eluted with the largest cell population.[27] Recently, however, it has been reported that a more primitive cell population may be distributed throughout the various fractions.[28] Table 9-3, demonstrates that the lymphocyte fractions are most enriched in the 70 mL/minute, 110 mL/minute, and 140 mL/minute fractions, while the majority of the clonogenic colony-forming units–granulocyte/macrophage (CFU-GM) activity is seen in the "rotor off" fraction. This excellent preparative technique can be combined with other selective techniques based on the phenotypic or immunologic criteria.

Lectin-Based Techniques

Several TCD techniques are based on an initial debulking and concentration step using either soluble or plastic-bound SBA.[29,30] Bone marrow is first subjected to a red blood cell (RBC) depletion

Table 9-3. Recovery of Necleated Cells, Lymphocytes and Hematopoietic Progenitor Cells From Fractions Collected by Counterflow Centrifugation Elutriation of Human Bone Marrow[27]

Fraction	Total Nucleated Cells* ($\times 10^9$)	Percent Lymphocytes*	Number CFU-GM* ($\times 10^6$)
Harvest	32.0 ± 1.1	16.2 ± 1.8	Not Done
Buffy coat	14.2 ± 0.6	20.3 ± 1.5	20.9 ± 9.0
70 mL/minute	5.0 ± 0.3	89.0 ± 1.8	3.6 ± 3.6
110 mL/minute	1.6 ± 0.1	50.9 ± 3.9	2.2 ± 1.2
140 mL/minute	0.9 ± 0.1	49.5 ± 5.6	0.9 ± 1.0
Rotor Off	6.7 ± 0.3	0.3 ± 0.1	13.0 ± 8.2

* Mean ± SD

step by Ficoll-Hypaque separation or to unit-gravity sedimentation with hydroxyethyl starch or gelatin. Then it is exposed to SBA, which binds selectively to all mature blood elements (RBCs, T cells, B cells, monocytes, granulocytes, stromal cells, and dendritic cells) via their N-acetyl-D-galactosamine residues, while not binding to hematopoietic progenitor cells. SBA– cells are separated from the SBA+ cells either on a 5% bovine serum albumin gradient or by lack of adherence to polystyrene-coupled SBA. This results in a concentration of progenitor cells and a 1 $\log_{10}$ depletion of T cells. The nonagglutinated or binding cells (SBA–) still contain enough T cells to induce GVHD, but they can easily be subjected to further TCD procedures.

The majority of lectin-separated transplants are performed by using rosetting with sheep erythrocytes for removal of residual T cells from the SBA– population. This standard cell preparative technique reproducibly reduces the T-cell content of the resultant SBA–E– graft to below that which causes GVHD in recipients of HLA-matched bone marrow recipients. Treatment with magnetic microspheres coupled to anti-T-cell MoAbs has also been used. Adherence on plastic to which anti-T-cell MoAbs have been covalently bound has been used in a series of clinical trials.[19] While comparative trials of different TCD methods are notably lacking in this field, some experimental data demonstrate that adequate TCD can be expected from combinations of these

Table 9-4. Comparison of T-Cell Depletion Methods

Treatment (N=3)	% E_{AET} Rosettes* (%)	Stimulation Index+	Depletion by LDA† ($\log_{10}$)
Untreated	17.1 ± 3.8	22.9 ± 7.2	
CP1 +C'	0.5 ± 0.5	1.2 ± 0.4	2.3 ± 0.2
XomaZyme-H65	28.0 ± 16.0	1.4 ± 0.4	2.0 ± 0.3
SBA–	9.0 ± 3.6	4.2 ± 0.8	1.3 ± 0.2
SBA–E–	0.1 ± 0.1	1.1 ± 0.2	2.9 ± 0.4
SBA–B–	0	1.0 ± 0.1	3.2 ± 0.3

* Values expressed as mean ± SEM.
+ Stimulation index = $\dfrac{\text{PHA–stimulated sample (cpm)}}{\text{unstimulated sample (cpm)}}$
† Limiting-dilution analysis; depletion calculated from starting sample.

techniques.[31] Table 9-4 presents the results from single marrow samples that have been T-cell-depleted by a variety of methods, including the MoAb CAMPATH plus complement, the ricin-A conjugated MoAb H-65 and SBA agglutination alone and combined with rosetting or treatment with immunomagnetic microspheres bearing the anti-T-cell MoAbs reactive with CD2, CD3 and CD8. SBA alone achieved the standard 1 $\log_{10}$ TCD, while the monoclonal techniques using CAMPATH and the immunotoxin showed a 2 $\log_{10}$ TCD. The highest overall depletion was achieved using the stepwise combination methods of initial SBA agglutination and either rosetting ($\log_{10}$ =2.9) or treatment with immunomagnetic microspheres ($\log_{10}$=3.2).

Defining Adequate Levels of T-Cell Depletion

A significant event in the understanding of the basis of the immunologic interaction in BMT in the clinical setting was the correlation of T-cell dose and the appearance of symptomatic GVHD. It was seen that the administration of grafts with more than 1×10^5 clonable T cells/kg resulted in Grade I or II GVHD in 50% of the recipients of HLA-matched grafts from family members.[21] Adequate levels of TCD will undoubtedly be dictated by the degree of disparity between donor and recipient. In grafts from unrelated donors, the threshold may well fall below this dose because of the effect of the increased number of mismatched minor histocompatibility antigens as compared to the family member situation.

The T-Cell Depletion Balance Sheet

In summary, the use of T-cell-depleted transplantation has resulted in significant reduction in GVHD and its complications in HLA-matched and -mismatched BMTs. The impact of this therapy can be seen most dramatically in the older transplant recipient and in recipients of matched, unrelated and partially matched, related bone marrow. Yet, TCD has also resulted in the problems of increased graft rejection or failure and, in some diseases, of increased posttransplant relapse rates. The development of diverse TCD methods has made comparison of clinical outcomes of laboratory manipulations difficult, but these methods have given tantalizing hints as to the function of T-cell populations in engraftment,

GVHD, graft-vs-leukemia effect and immunologic reconstitution. Further, increasingly sophisticated methods of cell subpopulation identification and separation indicate that true graft engineering, the construction of hematopoietic grafts with specific standard and desired characteristics, may be on the horizon.

References

1. O'Reilly RJ. T cell depletion and allogeneic bone marrow transplantation. Semin Hematol 1992;29(Suppl1):20-6.
2. Beatty PG, Hervé P. Immunogenetic factors relevant to human acute graft-versus-host disease. In: Burakoff SJ, Deeg HJ, Ferrara J, Atkinson K, eds. Graft-vs-host disease: Immunology, pathophysiology and treatment. New York, NY: Marcel Dekker, 1990:415-23.
3. Poynton C. Matching techniques and HLA typing. In: Treleaven J, Barrett J., eds. Bone marrow transplantation in practice. Edinburgh, UK: Churchill Livingstone, 1992:187-206.
4. Kaminski E, Sharrock C, Ilows J, et al. Frequency analysis of cytotoxic T lymphocyte precursors—possible relevance to HLA matched unrelated donor bone marrow transplantation. Bone Marrow Transplant 1988;3:149-65.
5. Schwarer A, Juang YZ, Brookes PA, et al. Frequency of antirecipient alloreactive helper T cell precursors in donor blood and graft-versus-host diseases after HLA-identical sibling bone marrow transplantation. Lancet 1993;341:203-5.
6. Deeg HJ, Cottler-Fox M. Clinical spectrum and pathophysiology of acute graft-versus-host disease. In: Burakoff SJ, Deeg HJ, Ferrara J, Atkinson K, eds. Graft-vs-host disease: Immunology, pathophysiology and treatment. New York, NY: Marcel Dekker, 1990:311-36.
7. Korngold R, Sprent J. Lethal graft-versus-host disease after bone marrow transplantation across minor histocompatibility barriers in mice: Prevention by removing mature T cells from marrow. J Exp Med 1978;148:1687-98.
8. Reisner Y, Kapoor N, Kirkpatrick D, et al. Transplantation for acute leukaemia with HLA-A and B nonidentical parental marrow cells fractionated with soybean agglutinin and sheep red cells. Lancet 1981;2:327-31.
9. Barrett J. Graft-versus-host diseases. In: Treleaven J, Barrett J, eds. Bone marrow transplantation in practice. Edinburgh, UK: Churchill Livingstone, 1992:257-69.

10. van Bekkum D. Graft-vs-host disease. In: van Bekkum D, Löwenberg B, eds. Bone marrrow transplantation: Biological mechanisms and clinical practice. New York, NY: Marcel Dekker, 1985:147-212.
11. Martin PJ, Kernan NA. T cell depletion for the prevention of graft-vs-host disease. In: Burakoff SJ, Deeg HJ, Ferrara J, Atkinson K, eds. Graft-vs-host disease: Immunology, pathophysiology and treatment. New York, NY: Marcel Dekker, 1990:371-87.
12. Kernan NA. Graft failure following transplantation of T cell depleted marrow. In: Burakoff SJ, Deeg HJ, Ferrara J, Atkinson K, eds. Graft-vs-host disease: Immunology, pathophysiology and treatment. New York, NY: Marcel Dekker, 1990:557-68.
13. Champlin R. Graft-versus-leukemia without graft-versus-host disease: An elusive goal of bone marrow transplantation. Semin Hematol 1992;3(Suppl2):46-51.
14. Kernan NA. T cell depletion for prevention of graft versus host disease. In: Forman SJ, Blume KG, Thomas ED, eds. Bone marrow transplantation. Cambridge, MA. Blackwell Scientific Publications. 1994:124-35.
15. Kernan NA, Bartsch G, Ash RC, et al. Analysis of 462 unrelated marrow transplants facilitated by the National Marrow Donor Program. N Engl J Med 1993;328:593-602.
16. Nemunaitis J, Buckner CD, Appelbaum FR, et al. Phase I/II trial of recombinant human granulocyte-macrophage colony stimulating factor following allogeneic bone marrow transplantation. Blood 1991;77:2065-71.
17. Collins N, Kernan NA, Bleau S, O'Reilly RJ. T cell depletion of allogeneic human bone marrow grafts by soybean lectin agglutination and either sheep red blood cell rosetting or adherence on the CD5/CD8 CELLector™. In: Gee AP, ed. Bone marrow processing and purging: A practical guide. Boca Raton, FL: CRC Press, 1991:201-12.
18. Bierer B. Evaluation of efficiency of T cell depletion. In: Areman EM, Deeg HJ, Sacher RA, eds. Bone marrow and stem cell processing: A manual of current techniques. Philadelphia, PA: F.A. Davis, 1992:430-5.
19. Collins NH, Carabasi MH, Bleau S, et al. New technology for the depletion of T cells from soybean lectin agglutinated, HLA-matched bone marrow grafts for leukemia: Initial laboratory and clinial results. In: Worthington-White DA, Gee

AP, Gross S, eds. Advances in bone marrow purging and processing. New York, NY: Wiley-Liss, 1992:427-39.

20. Kernan NA, Flomenberg N, Collins NH, et al. Quantitation of T lymphocytes in human bone marrow by a limiting dilution assay. Transplantation 1985;40:317-22.

21. Kernan NA, Collins NH, Juliano L, et al. Clonable T lymphocytes in T cell depleted bone marrow transplants correlate with development of graft-versus-host disease. Blood 1986,68:770-3.

22. Smith C, Gasparetto C, Collins N, et al. Purification and partial characterization of a human hematopoietic precursor population. Blood 1991;77:2122-8.

23. Carabasi MH, Collins NH, Papapdopoulos E, et al. New technology for depletion of T cells from soybean lectin agglutinated (SBA-), HLA-matched bone marrow grafts for leukemia: Initial clinical results (abstract). Blood 1991;78(Suppl1):225a.

24. Preti RA, Collins N, Gee A. ISHAGE bone marrow processing survey: Preliminary report on an international information gathering process. J Hematol 1993;2:103-9.

25. Marciniak E, Romond EH, Thompson JS, Henslee PJ. Laboratory control in predicting clinical efficacy of T cell depletion procedures used for prevention of graft-versus-host disease: Importance of limiting dilution analysis. Bone Marrow Transplant 1988;3:589-98.

26. Uckun F, Myers DE. Allograft and autograft purging using immunotoxins in clinical bone marrow transplantation for hematologic malignancies. J Hematol 1993:2:155-63.

27. Davis JM, Noga SJ, Thoburn CY, et al. Lymphocyte depletion of bone marow grafts using elutriation. In: Areman EM, Deeg HJ, Sacher RA, eds. Bone marrow and stem cell processing: A manual of current techniques. Philadelphia, PA: F.A. Davis, 1992:181-95.

28. Wagner JE, Lebkowski J, Fahey S, et al. Large-scale isolation of primitive human hematopoietic stem cells by counterflow elutriation (CE) and CD34+ selection (abstract). Blood 1992;80(Suppl1):921a.

29. Collins NH, Bleau S, Kernan NA, O'Reilly RJ. T cell depletion of bone marrow by treatment with soybean agglutinin and sheep red blood cell rosetting. In: Areman EM, Deeg HJ, Sacher, RA, eds. Bone marrow and stem cell processing: A

manual of current techniques. Philadelphia, PA: F.A. Davis, 1992:171-80.

30. Lebkowski JS, Schain LR, Okrongly D, et al. Rapid isolation of human CD34 hematopoietic stem cells—purging of human tumor cells. Transplantation 1992;53:1011-19.

31. Frame JN, Collins NH, Cartagena T, et al. T cell depletion of human bone marrow: Comparison of Campath-1 plus complement, anti-T-cell ricin A chain immunotoxin and soybean agglutinin alone or in combination with sheep erythrocytes or immunomagnetic beads. Transplantation 1989;47:984-8.

In: Lasky L and Warkentin P, eds. *Marrow and Stem Cell*
Processing for Transplantation
Bethesda, MD: American Association of Blood Banks, 1995

10

Peripheral Blood Stem Cells

Larry C. Lasky, MD

H EMATOPOIETIC PROGENITORS ARE PRESENT in the circulating blood as well as in the marrow. These progenitors can be used to promote hematopoietic recovery in marrow-depleted patients. This treatment modality is becoming widely accepted by clinicians who treat these critically ill patients.

History

Early experiments allowed identification of hematopoietic progenitors in peripheral blood. Cross-circulation studies, in which the use of healthy dogs could rescue lethally irradiated ones, showed that viable, probably pluripotent, progenitor cells circulate and can promote hematopoietic recovery.[1]

Early studies also showed that these cells are present in the circulation of humans and can be collected by apheresis.[2,3] The progenitors in the circulation have many of the same characteristics as seen in progenitors collected in marrow. Their size and density are similar,[4] as are their antigenic makeups.[5,6] However, mature erythroid and megakaryocytoid committed progenitors (CFU-E and CFU-Mk) are much less frequent in the circulation than their less committed counterparts (BFU-E and BFU-Mk), while in the marrow they are easily identified in quantity.[7]

It has been known for many years that chronic myelogenous leukemia (CML) cells collected during chronic phase can induce hematopoiesis, albeit abnormal hematopoiesis, when infused.

Larry C. Lasky, MD, Director, Division of Transfusion Medicine, Associate Professor, Departments of Pathology and Internal Medicine, Ohio State University, Columbus, Ohio

Two early clinical trials of the use of nonmalignant peripheral blood stem cells (PBSCs) in lieu of autologous or syngeneic marrow were unsuccessful, perhaps because of the low number of cells infused.[8,9] Two different successes were reported in this context in the 1980s. In one case, a father's PBSCs collected by apheresis were used in an attempt to cure the son's adenine deaminase (ADA)-deficient immune disorder.[10] The patient's ADA levels rose, but his red blood cells (RBCs) continued to have his own rather than his father's phenotype. In the secnd case, Storb and colleagues[11] reported using buffy coat collected from the marrow donor to avoid marrow rejection in aplastic anemia patients undergoing marrow transplant. The presence of hematopoietic progenitors in the buffy coats is one possible explanation for this protection from rejection. However, as would be expected from the presence of T cells in the buffy coats, graft-vs-host disease (GVHD) was more common in the patients receiving buffy coats.

Mobilization

Increasing the number of circulating progenitors increases the number that can be collected by apheresis. There are several means of intentionally increasing the number of progenitors in the circulation. One is diurnal variation, with a peak of committed progenitors in the afternoon about 50-100% higher than in the morning.[12] This diurnal variation can be reversed by the use of oral prednisone.[12] Exercise increases the number of circulating progenitors, as does a previous apheresis collection.[13-15] A number of substances also cause increased circulation of progenitors. These include endotoxin, folinic acid, corticotropin, and dextran.[16]

The most effective ways to promote the circulation of progenitors, and the ones that are used clinically, are chemotherapy and hematopoietic growth factors. As the marrow recovers from marrow-toxic therapy, the number of circulating progenitors increases markedly, by as much as a factor of 20.[17-26] Hematopoietic growth factors, notably the currently available granulocyte/macrophage colony-stimulating factor (GM-CSF) and granulocyte CSF (G-CSF) have a similar effect.[19,21,23,26-34] The combination of growth factors and chemotherapy is synergistic.

GM-CSF was the first growth factor observed to have the property of increasing the number of circulating hematopoietic progenitors. Socinski and colleagues[35] showed that GM-CSF alone or in combination with high-dose chemotherapy could have this effect. Subsequent studies showed that PBSCs collected from patients under these conditions had neutrophil recovery greatly increased in speed over that in patients treated with unstimulated PBSCs.[36]

G-CSF has subsequently been shown to have a similar effect, with potentially significant advantages. G-CSF not only increases the number of circulating progenitors and the speed with which these progenitors promote neutrophil recovery, but it causes increased speed of platelet recovery.[32] This can lead to fewer platelet transfusions, lower morbidity and mortality due to hemorrhage and quicker hospital discharge. Moreover, administration of G-CSF appears to cause fewer side effects than that of GM-CSF. While the former can cause a number of side effects, including capillary leak syndrome and pericarditis, toxicity of G-CSF is largely limited to bone pain and occasional flu-like symptoms (as are also seen with GM-CSF).

Collection Techniques

Machines

Essentially all of the blood cell separators that are used clinically to collect platelets and granulocytes have been used to collect PBSCs. These include the Fenwal CS-3000 (Baxter Healthcare Corporation, Deerfield, IL),[37-44] the Haemonetics Model V50 (Haemonetics Corporation, Braintree, MA),[2,37] and the COBE Spectra (COBE Laboratories, Lakewood, CO).[43-45] All have been demonstrated to be effective in collecting the desired progenitor cells. The machines differ in the degree of automation and the nature of the component collected. Some of the salient characteristics are volume, red cell content and leukocyte differential, including the granulocyte content. For a given machine, many or all of these characteristics can be adjusted by the operator, and may vary depending on features of the donor-patient. Some collection characteristics taken from published reports are shown in Table 10-1.

Vascular Access

Vascular access for collection of PBSCs is similar to that needed for any therapeutic apheresis procedure. If antecubital veins can

Table 10-1. Some Blood Cell Separator PBSC Collection Results

Machine	Number of Nucleated Cells Collected	Red Cell Content	% Neutrophils	Procedure Details	Reference
CS-3000	1×10^8/kg	5 mL	7	Two children, 3-hour collections	39
CS-3000	0.59×10^{10}	11 mL	32 (automated differential)	10 L Processed in 183 minutes	44
CS-3000	0.9×10^8/kg	Not given	Median 0 Range not given	7 L in 3 hours	56
COBE Spectra	0.77×10^{10}	8 mL	28 (automated differential)	10 L Processed in 143 minutes	44

be used, they are. However, very often, the antecubital veins are sclerosed as a result of chemotherapy and frequent blood drawing. In this case, central lines are used. Some problems with clotting of these lines have been reported.[46] This appears to be more of a problem with GM-CSF stimulation.[47]

Procedure Specification

The length, frequency and timing of PBSC collection procedures depend on many factors. These include features of the machine used, the patient and the therapeutic protocol.

Dose

The prime determinant of the nature and quantity of procedures to be used for collection is the desired dose of PBSCs to be used. In the absence of stimulation of circulating progenitors, most reports have described using doses of $6\text{-}10 \times 10^8$ nucleated cells per kilogram of patient mass. Mononuclear cells (lymphocytes and monocytes) ideally make up most or all of the nucleated cells in a PBSC collection. Several factors, including the machine and the procedure used, determine the precise percentage. Usually the mononuclear cell count approximates the nucleated cell count. If there is a high percentage of neutrophils in the collection, it may be wisest to use the mononuclear rather than the nucleated cell count in determining dose.

Using growth factor or chemotherapy mobilization of PBSCs, the best dosage parameter to use and the required level of this parameter are not as well-defined. Such mobilization increases the number of progenitors in a given number of nucleated or mononuclear cells in a way that is not always predictable. The most common alternatives to nucleated cell or mononuclear cell count that are cited in the literature are the number of colony-forming units–granulocyte/macrophage (CFU-GM) or the number of CD34+ cells. The problems with the former are several. It takes 2 weeks to perform a CFU-GM assay, which makes it difficult to use in the context of daily or even thrice weekly collections. The assay has a very large coefficient of variation even within a given laboratory, and interinstitutional variations in this measurement, even between patients receiving identical treatment, are immense. The other frequently used parameter, the number of CD34+ cells, is fairly difficult to measure in a precise and accurate way. These measurements are discussed thoroughly in Chapter 2. As a practical matter, we find that using a goal of 6×10^8 nucleated cells per kg works well from a collection viewpoint, as well as clinically, even with G-CSF-stimulated patients.

Frequency

Frequency is dictated more by the time relationship to mobilization than by any other consideration. If the collections are made to coincide with the peak of circulating progenitors following some mobilization maneuver, the wisest method is probably to perform daily collections to take advantage of that peak. An exception to this is the small patient in whom either the mononuclear cell count falls significantly or the platelet count falls dangerously during collection. In this case, collections may have to be spaced every other day or less often, depending on how fast the relevant count rises.

One can take extra measures to prevent a drop in platelet count. Large drops in platelet count, when seen, often occur in conjunction with the collection of large numbers of platelets.

With the Fenwal CS-3000, one can use the small-volume collection chamber, which allows more of the platelets to flow back into the patient (at the possible risk of losing some mononuclear cells). There may be an advantage to collecting more platelets at the time of PBSC apheresis, however. A protective effect of the cryopreserved platelets collected incidentally with the mononuclear cells in the PBSCs has been noted.[48] It appears that these platelets function in the patient after infusion.

Length

The length of the procedure is to some extent arbitrary, and it can be fit to the available facilities and personnel. However, in general the longer the procedure, the more progenitors are collected. The number of progenitors does not drop off with time in most cases. Our group has shown this for 3-hour collections on the Fenwal CS-3000.[49] Hillyer et al[15] have published data suggesting that the collection efficiency for hematopoietic progenitors actually increases during prolonged collections, at least in normal donors. Others have observed a drop in the number of circulating mononuclear cells (and presumably progenitors) in long procedures in very small children (10-20 kg), but not in larger children or adult patients.

PBSC Processing

Once PBSCs have been collected, they may need to be processed before cryopreservation. The two most common indications for such processing are high fluid volume and red cell content. Larger volumes mean more dimethylsulfoxide (DMSO) preservative and more volume infused to the patient after thawing. Simple centrifugation before freezing allows the removal of excess volume. The amount of supernatant fluid that can be removed is determined by the desired final cell concentration. This is usually 100 million nucleated cells per mL, although higher concentrations may be acceptable (Rowley S, personal communication). Any other procedure that lowers the number of irrelevant cells, such as CD34+ selection, will have the effect of lowering the volume to be infused after thawing.

Some blood cell separators, used with certain operating methods, collect a high number of RBCs with the PBSCs. Since RBCs tend to hemolyze during freezing and thawing by methods designed to preserve hematopoietic progenitor cells, and since these hemolyzed RBCs can cause disseminated intravascular coagulation and renal failure when infused in large quantities, it is best to minimize their numbers. This can be accomplished simply by centrifugation in bags or tubes to produce a buffy coat, which is retained. A buffy coat can also be obtained using a cell processor such as the COBE 2991 or a blood cell separator, such as the Fenwal CS-3000 or the Haemonetics Model V50 in an off-line mode (see Chapter 4).

A third possibility is discontinuous density-gradient centrifugation. The freezing-thawing procedure also does not preserve granulocytes. The ruptured remains of these cells may be responsible for some of the reactions observed in patients during infusion of PBSCs or marrow. Some authors have advocated a processing method that removes more than 99% of the RBCs and 95% of the granulocytes. This method is a discontinuous density-gradient centrifugation. The usual specific gravity of the support solution, which can be Ficoll-diatrizoate or Percoll, is approximately 1.077. Centrifugation can be carried out in a simple refrigerated centrifuge, or it can be done in a blood processor (eg, the COBE 2991) or a blood cell separator.

In an allogeneic setting, one may also wish to remove T cells. Dooley and colleagues[50] have described a method of removing T cells using sheep RBCs and a discontinuous Percoll density-gradient centrifugation. This method was used in a case report of allogeneic transplantation with PBSCs.[51]

PBSCs may contain fewer malignant cells than marrow from the same patient, especially when the marrow is known to be positive for tumor cells. For instance, in neuroblastoma, Moss and colleagues have shown that marrow is much more often involved than are PBSCs collected from the same patients, although malignant cells can occasionally be detected in the PBSC collections.[52] For this reason, purging of malignant cells may be necessary as (or if) it is for marrow used in the autologous setting. Similar methods as are used for marrow may be used. (See Chapters 6, 7 and 8.) Positive selection, as discussed in Chapter 13, may be an alternative to the removal of malignant cells. Similar methods would be used.

In-vitro expansion of progenitor cells, as described in Chapter 12, may allow collection of relatively few PBSCs that will have the same effect as larger or more numerous collections. This may also allow purging of smaller volumes of cells in advance of expansion. Expansion may be directed at normal rather than malignant progenitors, allowing the in-vitro expansion to accomplish the removal of malignant cells. In-vitro expansion also may allow repeated clinical use of a single or limited numbers of collections of PBSCs, allowing multiple cycles of intensive radio-chemotherapy.

Clinical Applications

Indications

The most reported use for PBSCs initially was in acute nonlymphocytic leukemia (ANLL). Many reports have described using PBSCs collected in the recovery phase after chemotherapy in ANLL, as the patient goes into remission. The autograft is most frequently performed, and is most successful, in remission. There is some evidence that the probability of malignant progenitors in the circulation is lower as the patient goes into remission.[53] Performing PBSC harvest at this time also maximizes the number of circulating progenitors, since the number increases dramatically as the white blood cell count and platelet count rebound following induction chemotherapy.[54] Körbling and colleagues[55] reported a study comparing mafosfamide-treated autologous marrow to PBSCs as a source of cellular support following total-body irradiation and high-dose cyclophosphamide in acute myelogenous leukemia patients in first complete remission. There were 23 patients in the marrow group and 20 in the PBSC group. Hematopoietic recovery was significantly faster in the PBSC group, as one would expect, if only because of the delay caused by mafosfamide treatment of the marrow. Probability of 2-year disease-free survival was 51% in the marrow group and 35% in the PBSC group, although the difference was not statistically significant.

Lymphoma, both Hodgkin's and non-Hodgkin's, currently rivals ANLL for the most reported application of PBSCs. In 1989, this author and colleagues[56] published a controlled but not randomized study of PBSCs vs marrow as a source of cells for rescue following marrow-toxic chemotherapy in refractory Hodgkin's disease patients. In six of seven PBSC-treated patients, they were selected to receive PBSCs because their marrow was involved with disease. Hematopoietic recovery and hospital discharge following infusion of the cells was more rapid in the PBSC group than in the marrow-treated group. PBSCs were not mobilized with chemotherapy or growth factors in this early study. However, five of the six patients treated with PBSCs because of marrow involvement developed recurrent disease. This may have been due to the underlying aggressiveness of the disease in these patients and the inability of the preparative regimen to eradicate it. Another possibility is the presence of malignant progenitor cells in the collected PBSCs.

Kessinger and colleagues[57] reported an actuarial 18-month survival of 15% in 16 patients with refractory Hodgkin's disease treated with unstimulated PBSCs. These patients were treated with PBSCs rather than marrow for a variety of reasons, including marrow involvement. In a German study, patients were treated with PBSCs because their iliac crests had been irradiated in the course of primary treatment. Seven of 11 evaluable patients were alive and in unmaintained complete remission at a median of 318 days.[58] Kessinger and colleagues[59] published a follow-up report of 56 patients with relapsed Hodgkin's disease treated with PBSCs, with an overall actuarial 3-year survival of 37%. The 30 patients who had not had marrow involvement at the time of PBSC harvest had an actuarial event-free survival of 47%.[59]

The treatment of choice for relapsed aggressive lymphoma appears to be high-dose radiochemotherapy followed by cellular support in the form of marrow or PBSCs.[60] An argument can be made that such therapy may be warranted and effective as primary treatment for some forms of lymphoma.[60] There are data that, although morphologically lymphoma-free marrow may often contain clonogenic malignant cells, this is less likely to be true with PBSC collections.[61] In a recent report, Dreyfus and colleagues described autografting with PBSCs to treat high-risk non-Hodgkin's lymphoma.[62] They achieved a 37% 2-year actuarial disease-free survival.

CML is another of the first reported applications of PBSCs. Indeed, it was one of the areas in which the idea of cellular rescue following marrow-toxic therapy was pioneered. A case report of autografting in CML with PBSCs carried out soon after diagnosis leading to Philadelphia chromosome-negative normal hematopoiesis more than 2 years after transplant appeared in 1987.[63] In a study of 14 CML patients autografted with PBSCs in chronic phase, two patients had "predominantly Ph-negative hematopoiesis" approximately 4 years after treatment.[64] In 47 cases of CML transplanted in transformation with autologous PBSCs, 43 entered a second chronic phase.[65] Most patients had recurrent transformation 2-43 months after transplant. Eight were alive in a second chronic phase a median of 24 months after transplant. When the treatment consisted of double transplant followed by alpha-interferon treatment, the second chronic phase lasted a median of 18 months.

A few reports have appeared discussing the use of PBSCs in acute lymphoblastic leukemia.[66-70] The advantages and disadvantages of using PBSCs vs marrow are not yet clear from the small number of transplants reported.

Solid tumors have been treated with autologous marrow transplantation, and PBSC transplant has been applied in this area as well. Breast cancer is by far the most frequently treated malignancy in this category. Kessinger and colleagues[71] reported rescuing two patients with breast cancer with unstimulated PBSCs. They concluded that this modality could be considered in lieu of autologous marrow if marrow could not be harvested. Since that report, PBSCs have been used either alone or with marrow in patients whose marrow was at least theoretically available.[30] For instance, Elias and colleagues reported treating 16 breast cancer patients with PBSCs following intensive chemotherapy.[23] These patients were treated with GM-CSF and cyclic chemotherapy prior to PBSC harvest. All had rapid hematopoietic recovery except for three patients who were given backup autologous marrow for delayed platelet recovery. These three patients had been heavily treated and had recovered slowly from previous chemotherapy. The authors felt that using PBSCs has the potential benefit of less time at risk of mortality and morbidity, and they may lower the cost of autologous transplant, compared to the use of marrow.

Solid tumors of childhood, especially neuroblastoma, have been treated with PBSCs. Neuroblastoma represents an especially compelling situation in which PBSCs may be useful, since patients with advanced neuroblastoma have marrow involvement. Our studies have shown that the peripheral blood is involved much less frequently than the marrow.[52] The main problem in using PBSCs is a technical one of collecting them from very small patients. We and others have reported doing this.[39,42,69] The major technical problems involved in such collections are those of extracorporeal volume and citrate toxicity. The former can be overcome by priming the machine with RBCs, with or without plasma or a colloid solution to avoid volume shifts. Citrate toxicity can be avoided or minimized by lowering the amount of citrate that is infused, primarily by substituting heparin for it.[42] Given that such PBSC transplants can be performed technically, the remaining problem is that of eradicating the neoplasm from the patient before infusing the rescuing cells. This is still being addressed.

Other tumors that have been treated with or considered for therapy with autologous PBSCs for hematopoietic rescue include lung,[33,72] germ cell,[73,74] ovarian[75] and Ewing's sarcoma.[76] The use of PBSCs to treat multiple myeloma is also being explored.[77-81]

Methods

A variety of strategies are possible for the clinical use of PBSCs. Among these are the use of unstimulated PBSCs, PBSCs mobilized with cytokines or chemotherapy, PBSCs used along with marrow and the combination of PBSCs with adoptive immunotherapy. Early clinical PBSC studies were performed with unmobilized cells, so-called steady-state PBSCs. When it was discovered that the number of progenitors could be increased by orders of magnitude in circulation and hence in the number of collected progenitors with the use of growth factors or chemotherapy, most clinical applications incorporated one or both of these modalities. Since it was suggested, largely before the use of growth factor mobilization, that occasional failure of hematopoietic recovery could occur following PBSC rescue alone, PBSCs have been combined in some studies with marrow.[28,76,82,83] This strategy combines the speed of recovery engendered by the PBSCs and the durability of recovery from the marrow. In fact, with growth-factor-expanded PBSCs, the addition of marrow may not be necessary.

Since PBSC collections contain a large number of lymphocytes, a possible future application of PBSCs is to manipulate these incidental lymphocytes so that they have a direct effect against the patient's malignancy. The PBSC collection would then provide ammunition against malignancy while promoting hematopoietic recovery.

Another future possibility for use of PBSCs is in allogeneic transplantation. The studies by Storb and colleagues[11] suggested that buffy coats helped reduce graft failure when used with marrow in allogeneic transplant for patients with aplastic anemia. Kessinger and colleagues[51] reported on an allogeneic transplant performed with T-cell-depleted PBSCs in a patient with acute lymphoblastic leukemia. Trilineage hematopoietic engraftment occurred, but the patient died too early for evaluation of GVHD or permanent engraftment.

Russell[84] recently reported a case of HLA-identical sibling transplantation for acute lymphoblastic leukemia in second complete remission using G-CSF-moiblized PBSCs. The donor was an obese, heavy smoker, which made marrow harvest difficult. No T-cell depletion was performed. Hematopoietic recovery time, except for platelet recovery, was comparable to marrow, not faster as one might expect with G-CSF-mobilized cells. Platelet recovery was prolonged, possibly as a result of moderate hepatic veno-occlusive disease. At 58 days (the time of the report), GVHD had not developed. The routine use of PBSCs for allogeneic transplant is a possibility in the future in cases where marrow is difficult to obtain, and perhaps in other settings such as use of an unrelated donor.

Results

In general, clinical outcome with respect to disease-free survival is similar whether PBSCs or marrow is used as the source of cellular support following marrow-lethal radiochemotherapy. Kessinger and colleagues[85] have presented preliminary data in lymphoma patients suggesting a *better* disease survival in patients given PBSCs, because of marrow involvement or unavailability, than in patients autografted with marrow. This suggestion that PBSCs may be superior to marrow has a couple of possible explanations. It may be that the lymphocytes and/or monocytes collected in vast abundance with the hematopoietic progenitors per se may have an effect in fighting the neoplasm. Perhaps more rapid immunologic recovery seen with PBSCs allows the patient to more successfully overcome the neoplasm.

Summary

It is now well-established that PBSCs can be used in lieu of marrow to promote autologous hematopoietic recovery following marrow-toxic chemoradiotherapy. The cells can be collected with a variety of apheresis equipment. Processing the cells for cryopreservation can be minimal, or the more complicated methods under development for positive selection or in-vitro expansion of marrow-derived progenitors may be applicable. Clinically, patients recover faster than if given marrow, especially with in-vivo growth factor or chemotherapy-expanded progenitors. Freedom from disease recurrence seems to be as good as and perhaps better than, if marrow is used.

Note: A number of excellent reviews covering various aspects of collection and use of PBSCs have been published. This author recommends them as a source of more or different detail for the interested reader.[5,60,75,86-94]

References

1. Epstein RB, Graham TC, Buckner CD, et al. Allogeneic marrow engraftment by cross circulation in lethally irradiated dogs. Blood 1966;28:692-707.
2. Weiner RS, Richman CM, Yankee RA. Semicontinuous flow centrifugation for the pheresis of immunocompetent cells and stem cells. Blood 1977;49:391-7.
3. Nguyen BT, Perkins HA. Quantitation of granulocyte-macrophage progenitor cells (CFU-C) in plateletpheresis and leukapheresis concentrates. Rev Fr Transfus Immunohematol 1979;22:489-500.
4. Lasky LC, Zanjani ED. Size and density characterization of human committed and multipotent hematopoietic progenitors. Exp Hematol 1985;13:680-4.
5. Silvestri F, Banavali S, Baccarani M, Preisler HD. The CD34 hemopoietic progenitor cell associated antigen: Biology and clinical applications. Haematologica 1992;77:265-73.
6. Udomsakdi C, Lansdorp PM, Hogge DE, et al. Characterization of primitive hematopoietic cells in normal human peripheral blood. Blood 1992;80:2513-21.
7. Zauli G, Vitale L, Brunelli MA, Bagnara GP. Prevalence of the primitive megakaryocyte progenitors (BFU-meg) in adult human peripheral blood. Exp Hematol 1992;20:850-4.
8. Abrams RA, Glaubiger D, Appelbaum FR, Deisseroth AB. Result of attempted hematopoietic reconstitution using isologous, peripheral blood mononuclear cells: A case report. Blood 1980;56:516-20.

9. Hershko C, Gale RP, Ho WG, Cline MJ. Cure of aplastic anemia in paroxysmal nocturnal haemoglobinuria by marrow transfusion from identical twin: Failure of peripheral-leukocyte transfusion to correct marrow aplasia. Lancet 1979;1:945-7.

10. Rich KC, Richman CM, Mejias E, Daddona P. Immunoreconstitution by peripheral blood leukocytes in adenosine deaminase-deficient severe combined immunodeficiency. J Clin Invest 1980;66:389-95.

11. Storb R, Doney KC, Thomas ED. Marrow transplantation with or without donor buffy coat cells for 65 transfused aplastic anemia patients. Blood 1982;59:236-46.

12. Lasky LC, Ascensao J, McCullough J, Zanjani ED. Steroid modulation of naturally occurring diurnal variation in circulating pluripotential haematopoietic cells (CFU-GEMM). Br J Haematol 1983;55:615-22.

13. Heal JM, Brightman A. Exercise and circulating hematopoietic progenitor cells (CFU-GM) in humans. Transfusion 1987;27:115-8.

14. Abboud CN, Brennan JK, Lichtman MA, Nusbacher J. Quantification of erythroid and granulocytic precursor cells in plateletpheresis residues. Transfusion 1980;20:9-16.

15. Hillyer CD, Tiegerman KO, Berkman EM. Increase in circulating colony-forming units–granulocyte-macrophage during large-volume leukapheresis: Evaluation of a new cell separator. Transfusion 1991;31:327-32.

16. Laporte JP, Douay L, Allieri A, et al. Expansion by folinic acid of the peripheral blood progenitor pool after chemotherapy: Its use in autografting in acute leukaemia. Br J Haematol 1990;74:445-51.

17. Kotasek D, Shepherd KM, Sage RE, et al. Factors affecting blood stem cell collections following high-dose cyclophosphamide mobilization in lymphoma, myeloma and solid tumors. Bone Marrow Transplant 1992;9:11-17.

18. Craig JIO, Smith SM, Parker AC, Anthony RS. The response of peripheral blood stem cells to standard chemotherapy for lymphoma. Leuk Lymphoma 1992;6:363-8.

19. Brugger W, Bross K, Frisch J, et al. Mobilization of peripheral blood progenitor cells by sequential administration of interleukin-3 and granulocyte-macrophage colony-stimulating factor following polychemotherapy with etoposide, ifosfamide, and cisplatin. Blood 1992;79:1193-200.

20. Fukuda M, Kojima S, Matsumoto K, Matsuyama T. Autotransplantation of peripheral blood stem cells mobilized by chemotherapy and recombinant human granulocyte colony-stimulating factor in childhood neuroblastoma and non-Hodgkin's lymphoma. Br J Haematol 1992;80:327-31.

21. Demuynck H, Pettengell R, De Campos E, et al. The capacity of peripheral blood stem cells mobilised with chemotherapy plus G-CSF to repopulate irradiated marrow stroma in vitro is similar to that of bone marrow. Eur J Cancer 1992;28:381-6.

22. Huan SD, Hester J, Spitzer G, et al. Influence of mobilized peripheral blood cells on the hematopoietic recovery by autologous marrow and recombinant human granulocyte-macrophage colony-stimulating factor after high-dose cyclophosphamide, etoposide, and cisplatin. Blood 1992;79:3388-93.

23. Elias AD, Ayash L, Anderson KC, et al. Mobilization of peripheral blood progenitor cells by chemotherapy and granulocyte-macrophage colony-stimulating factor for hematologic support after high-dose intensification for breast cancer. Blood 1992;79:3036-44.

24. Ikematsu W, Teshima T, Kondo S, et al. Circulating CD34+ hematopoietic progenitors in the harvesting peripheral blood stem cells: Enhancement by recombinant human granulocyte colony-stimulating factor. Biotherapy 1992;5:131-6.

25. Bender JG, Williams SF, Myers S, et al. Characterization of chemotherapy mobilized peripheral blood progenitor cells for use in autologous stem cell transplantation. Bone Marrow Transplant 1992;10:281-5.

26. DeLuca E, Sheridan WP, Watson D, et al. Prior chemotherapy does not prevent effective mobilisation by G-CSF of peripheral blood progenitor cells. Br J Cancer 1992;66:893-9.

27. Tarella C, Ferrero D, Bregni M, et al. Peripheral blood expansion of early progenitor cells after high-dose cyclophosphamide and rhGM-CSF. Eur J Cancer 1991;27:22-7.

28. Gianni AM, Bregni M, Siena S, et al. Very rapid and complete hematopoietic reconstitution following combined transplantation of autologous bone marrow and GM-CSF-exposed stem cells. Bone Marrow Transplant 1991;4(Suppl 2):78.

29. Ho AD, Haas R, Korbling M, et al. Utilization of recombinant human GM-CSF to enhance peripheral progenitor cell yield for autologous transplantation. Bone Marrow Transplant 1991;7(Suppl 1):13-17.
30. Elias AD, Mazanet R, Wheeler C, et al. GM-CSF potentiated peripheral blood progenitor cell (PBPC) collection with or without bone marrow as hematologic support of high-dose chemotherapy: Two protocols. Breast Cancer Res Treat 1991;20(Suppl):S25-S29.
31. Antman KH. G-CSF and GM-CSF in clinical trials. Yale J Biol Med 1990;63:387-410.
32. Sheridan WP, Begley CG, Juttner CA, et al. Effect of peripheral-blood progenitor cells mobilised by filgrastim (G-CSF) on platelet recovery after high-dose chemotherapy. Lancet 1992;339:640-4.
33. Mukai J, Shimizu E, Ogura T. Granulocyte-colony-stimulating factor enhances the circulating hematopoietic progenitors in lung cancer patients treated with cisplatin-containing regimens. Jpn J Cancer Res 1992;83:746-53.
34. Teshima T, Harada M, Takamatsu Y, et al. Cytotoxic drug and cytotoxic drug/G-CSF mobilization of peripheral blood stem cells and their use for autografting. Bone Marrow Transplant 1992;10:215-20.
35. Socinski MA, Elias A, Schnipper L, et al. Granulocyte-macrophage colony stimulating factor expands the circulating haemopoietic progenitor cell compartment in man. Lancet 1988;1:1194-8.
36. Gianni AM, Siena S, Bregni M, Bonadonna G. The use of GM-CSF and peripheral blood stem cells (PBSC) minimises haematological toxicity following a myeloablative course of chemo-radiotherapy. Pathol Biol (Paris) 1992;39:956.
37. Kessinger A, Armitage JO, Landmark JD, et al. Autologous peripheral hematopoietic stem cell transplantation restores hematopoietic function following marrow ablative therapy. Blood 1988;71:723-7.
38. Lasky LC, Ash RC, Kersey JH, et al. Collection of pluripotential hematopoietic stem cells by cytapheresis. Blood 1982;59:822-7.
39. Lasky LC, Bostrom B, Smith J, et al. Clinical collection and use of peripheral blood stem cells in pediatric patients. Transplantation 1989;47:613-6.

40. To LB, Haylock DN, Thorp D, et al. The optimization of collection of peripheral blood stem cells for autotransplantation in acute myeloid leukaemia. Bone Marrow Transplant 1989;4:41-7.
41. Haylock D, Thorp D, To L, et al. Assessing the stem cell collection efficiency of the Fenwal CS3000. Prog Clin Biol Res 1990;337:67-9.
42. Lasky LC, Fox SB, Smith JA, Bostrom B. Collection and use of peripheral blood stem cells in very small pediatric patients. Bone Marrow Transplant 1991;7:281-4.
43. Craig JI, Anthony RS, Smith SM, et al. Comparison of the Cobe Spectra and Baxter CS3000 Cell Separators for the collection of peripheral blood stem cells from patients with hematological malignancies. Int J Cell Cloning 1992;10(Suppl 1):82-4.
44. Padley D, Strauss RG, Wieland M, Randels MJ. Concurrent comparison of the Cobe Spectra and Fenwal CS3000 for the collection of peripheral blood mononuclear cells for autologous peripheral blood stem cell transplantation. J Clin Apheresis 1991;6:77-80.
45. Norol F, Scotto F, Beaujean F, Duedari N. Optimization of peripheral blood stem cell (pbsc) collection procedure on a new apheresis device Spectra (Cobe*). Int J Cell Cloning 1992;10 (Suppl 1):196.
46. Haire WD, Lieberman RP, Lund GB, et al. Thrombotic complications of silicone rubber catheters during autologous marrow and peripheral stem cell transplantation: Prospective comparison of Hickman and Groshong catheters. Bone Marrow Transplant 1991;7:57-9.
47. Stephens LC, Haire WD, Schmit-Pokorny K, et al. Granulocyte macrophage colony stimulating factor: High incidence of apheresis catheter thrombosis during peripheral stem cell collection. Bone Marrow Transplant 1993;11:51-4.
48. Comenzo RL, Malachowski ME, Miller KB, et al. Engraftment with peripheral blood stem cells collected by large-volume leukapheresis for patients with lymphoma. Transfusion 1992;32:729-31.
49. Lasky LC, Smith JA, McCullough J, Zanjani ED. Three-hour collection of committed and multipotent hematopoietic progenitor cells by apheresis. Transfusion 1987;27:276-8.

50. Dooley DC, Law P, Alsop P. A new density gradient for the separation of large quantities of rosette-positive and rosette-negative cells. Exp Hematol 1987;15:296-303.

51. Kessinger A, Smith DM, Strandjord SE, et al. Allogeneic transplantation of blood-derived, T cell-depleted hemopoietic stem cells after myeloablative treatment in a patient with acute lymphoblastic leukemia. Bone Marrow Transplant 1989;4:643-6.

52. Moss TJ, Sanders DG, Lasky LC, Bostrom B. Contamination of peripheral blood stem cell harvests by circulating neuroblastoma cells. Blood 1990;76:1879-83.

53. To LB, Russell J, Moore S, Juttner CA. Residual leukemia cannot be detected in very early remission peripheral blood stem cell collections in acute non-lymphoblastic leukemia. Leuk Res 1987;11:327-9.

54. Cantin G, Marchand-Laroche D, Bouchard M, Leblond P. Blood-derived stem cell collection in acute nonlymphoblastic leukemia: Predictive factors for a good yield. Exp Hematol 1989;17:991-6.

55. Körbling M, Fliedner TM, Holle R, et al. Autologous blood stem cell (ABSCT) versus purged bone marrow transplantation (pABMT) in standard risk AML: Influence of source and cell composition of the autograft on hemopoietic reconstitution and disease-free survival. Bone Marrow Transplant 1991;7:343-9.

56. Lasky LC, Hurd DD, Smith JA, Haake R. Peripheral blood stem cell collection and use in Hodgkin's disease: Comparison with marrow in autologous transplantation. Transfusion 1989;29:323-7.

57. Kessinger A, Armitage JO, Smith DM, et al. High-dose therapy and autologous peripheral blood stem cell transplantation for patients with lymphoma. Blood 1989;74:1260-5.

58. Körbling M, Holle R, Haas R, et al. Autologous blood stem-cell transplantation in patients with advanced Hodgkin's disease and prior radiation to the pelvic site. J Clin Oncol 1990;8:978-85.

59. Kessinger A, Bierman PJ, Vose JM, Armitage JO. High-dose cyclophosphamide, carmustine, and etoposide followed by autologous peripheral stem cell transplantation for patients with relapsed Hodgkin's disease. Blood 1991;77:2322-5.

60. Urba WJ, Duffey PL, Longo DL. Treatment of patients with aggressive lymphomas: An overview. Monogr Natl Cancer Inst 1990;10:29-37.

61. Sharp JG, Joshi SS, Bierman P, et al. Significance of detection of occult non-Hodgkin's lymphoma in histologically uninvolved bone marrow by a culture technique. Blood 1992;79:1074-80.

62. Dreyfus F, Leblond V, Belanger C, et al. Peripheral blood stem cell collection and autografting in high risk lymphomas. Bone Marrow Transplant 1992;10:409-13.

63. Brito-Babapulle F, Apperley JF, Rassool F, et al. Complete remission after autografting for chronic myeloid leukaemia. Leuk Res 1987;11:1115-7.

64. Brito-Babapulle F, Bowcock SJ, Marcus RE, et al. Autografting for patients with chronic myeloid leukaemia in chronic phase: Peripheral blood stem cells may have a finite capacity for maintaining haemopoiesis. Br J Haematol 1989;73:76-81.

65. Reiffers J, Trouette R, Marit G, et al. Autologous blood stem cell transplantation for chronic granulocytic leukaemia in transformation: A report of 47 cases. Br J Haematol 1991;77:339-45.

66. Henon P, Debecker A, Lepers M, et al. Hemopoietic and immune reconstitution following peripheral blood stem cell autografting in acute leukemia (letter). Bone Marrow Transplant 1988;3:171-2.

67. Tilly H, Bastit D, Lucet JC, et al. Haemopoietic reconstitution after autologous peripheral blood stem cell transplantation in acute leukaemia (letter). Lancet 1986;2:154-5.

68. Watanabe T, Takaue Y, Kawano Y, et al. Peripheral blood stem cell autotransplantation in treatment of childhood cancer. Bone Marrow Transplant 1989;4:261-5.

69. Takaue Y, Watanabe T, Abe T, et al. Experience with peripheral blood stem cell collection for autografts in children with active cancer. Bone Marrow Transplant 1992;10:241-8.

70. Abe T, Koyama T, Takaue Y, et al. Successful autograft with peripheral blood stem cells in a child with T- lymphoblastic leukemia. Am J Pediatr Hematol Oncol 1992;14:66-9.

71. Kessinger A, Armitage JO, Landmark JD, Weisenburger DD. Reconstitution of human hematopoietic function with autologous cryopreserved circulating stem cells. Exp Hematol 1986;14:192-6.

72. Stiff PJ, Koester AR, Eagleton LE, et al. Autologous stem cell transplantation using peripheral blood stem cells. Transplantation 1987;44:585-8.

73. Beyer J, Grabbe J, Lenz K, et al. Cutaneous toxicity of high-dose carboplatin, etoposide and ifosfamide followed by autologous stem cell reinfusion. Bone Marrow Transplant 1992;10:491-4.

74. Bokemeyer C, Schmoll HJ. Treatment of advanced germ cell tumours by dose intensified chemotherapy with haematopoietic growth factors or peripheral blood stem cells (PBSC). Eur Urol 1993;23:223-9.

75. Panici PB, Scambia G, Baiocchi G, et al. Rationale for very high-dose chemotherapy with peripheral blood stem cell support in advanced ovarian cancer. Haematologica 1990;75 (Suppl 1):87-9.

76. Lopez M, Pouillart P, Du Puy Montbrun MC, et al. Fast hematological reconstitution after combined infusion of autologous bone marrow purged with mafosfamide and autologous peripheral blood stem cells in a patient with Ewing sarcoma (letter). Bone Marrow Transplant 1988;3:172-4.

77. Henon P, Beck G, Debecker A, et al. Autograft using peripheral blood stem cells collected after high dose melphalan in high risk multiple myeloma (letter). Br J Haematol 1988;70:254-5.

78. Fermand JP, Levy Y, Gerota J, et al. Treatment of aggressive multiple myeloma by high-dose chemotherapy and total body irradiation followed by blood stem cells autologous graft. Blood 1989;73:20-3.

79. Gianni AM, Tarella C, Siena S, et al. Durable and complete hematopoietic reconstitution after autografting of rhGM-CSF exposed peripheral blood progenitor cells. Bone Marrow Transplant 1990;6:143-5.

80. Fermand JP, Chevret S, Levy Y, et al. The role of autologous blood stem cells in support of high-dose therapy for multiple myeloma. Hematol Oncol Clin North Am 1992;6:451-62.

81. Jagannath S, Vesole DH, Glenn L, et al. Low-risk intensive therapy for multiple myeloma with combined autologous bone marrow and blood stem cell support. Blood 1992;80:1666-72.

82. Gianni AM, Bregni M, Siena S, et al. Rapid and complete hemopoietic reconstitution following combined transplan-

tation of autologous blood and bone marrow cells. A changing role for high dose chemo-radiotherapy? Hematol Oncol 1989;7:139-48.

83. Lopez M, Mortel O, Pouillart P, et al. Acceleration of hemopoietic recovery after autologous bone marrow transplantation by low doses of peripheral blood stem cells. Bone Marrow Transplant 1991;7:173-81.

84. Russell NH, Hunter A, Rogers S, et al. Peripheral blood stem cells as an alternative to marrow for allogeneic transplantation. Lancet 1993;341:1482.

85. Vose JM, Bierman PJ, Anderson JR, et al. High-dose chemotherapy with hematopoietic stem cells rescue for non-Hodgkin's lymphoma (NHL): Evaluation of event-free survival based on histologic subtype and rescue product (abstract). Proc Am Soc Clin Oncol 1992;11:318.

86. Juttner CA, To LB, Haylock DN, Dyson PG. Peripheral blood stem cell selection, collection and auto-transplantation. Prog Clin Biol Res 1990;333:447-59.

87. To LB, Juttner CA. Peripheral blood stem cell autografting: A new therapeutic option for AML. Br J Haematol 1987;66:285-8.

88. Bell AJ, Hamblin TJ, Oscier DG. Peripheral blood stem cell autografting. Hematol Oncol 1987;5:45-55.

89. Bensinger WI, Berenson RJ. Peripheral blood and positive selection of marrow as a source of stem cells for transplantation. Prog Clin Biol Res 1990;337:93-8.

90. Kessinger A, Armitage JO. The evolving role of autologous peripheral stem cell transplantation following high-dose therapy for malignancies. Blood 1991;77:211-3.

91. Kessinger A. Autologous transplantation with peripheral blood stem cells: A review of clinical results. J Clin Apheresis 1990;5:97-9.

92. Craig JIO, Turner ML, Parker AC. Peripheral blood stem cell transplantation. Blood Rev 1992;6:59-67.

93. Lowry PA, Tabbara IA. Peripheral hematopoietic stem cell transplantation: Current concepts. Exp Hematol 1992;20:937-42.

94. Kessinger A. Utilization of peripheral blood stem cells in autotransplantation. Hematol Oncol Clin North Am 1993;7:535-45.

In: Lasky L and Warkentin P, eds. *Marrow and Stem Cell Processing for Transplantation*
Bethesda, MD: American Association of Blood Banks, 1995

11

Human Umbilical Cord and Placental Blood Transplantation

Hal E. Broxmeyer, PhD

HEMATOPOIETIC CELLS CIRCULATING IN blood and found in other tissue areas are produced by stem and progenitor cells.[1,2] In the adult, the primary source of hematopoietic stem and progenitor cells is the bone marrow, which is the usual cellular choice for hematopoietic reconstitution in an autologous or major histocompatibility complex (MHC)-matched allogeneic setting.[3] Peripheral blood cells have also been used as a source of transplantable stem and progenitor cells.[4] However, this source of cells has been used mainly in the autologous situation. In this latter context, because of the very low frequency of progenitor cells in unperturbed blood, these cells are usually collected from blood after the patient has been conditioned with chemotherapy and/or infused with colony-stimulating factors (CSFs), such as granulocyte/macrophage CSF (GM-CSF), granulocyte CSF (G-CSF) and interleukin 3 (IL-3). At this time, the progenitor cells in blood are present in a higher frequency. It is not yet clear if blood truly contains long-term marrow repopulating cells. Ontologically, stem and progenitor cells are found first in the yolk sac, later in fetal liver and spleen, and then in fetal bone marrow.[5] To a more limited extent, fetal liver cells have also been used as a source of transplantable stem/progenitor cells.[6,7] It is not clear how stem and progenitor

Hal E. Broxmeyer, PhD, Departments of Medicine (Hematology/Oncology) and Microbiology/Immunology, and the Walther Oncology Center, Indiana University School of Medicine, Indianapolis, Indiana
(These studies were supported by Public Health Service Grants R37 CA36464, R01 HL46549 and R01 HL49202 from the National Institutes of Health and the National Cancer Institute.)

cells migrate,[8] but clinical medicine is already the beneficiary of this process.

A viable alternative to bone marrow as a source of hematopoietic progenitor cells is human umbilical cord blood,[9] which contains these cells in relatively high frequency as assessed by in-vitro colony assays. This includes stem cells, colony-forming units–granulocyte/macrophage (CFU-GM), burst-forming units–erythroid (BFU-E), CFU-megakaryocyte (CFU-MK) and multipotential CFU (CFU-GEMM) progenitor cells, as well as erythroid precursor cells [proerythroblast (CFU-E)]. Although the concentration of myeloid progenitor cells (MPCs) is elevated in the blood of newborn children for weeks after birth compared to that found in adult blood, by 1 day after birth the circulating concentration of MPC/mL is only 22-49% of that found in the cord blood of these same infants.[10] The collection of cord blood has been described in a greater detail.[9,11]

Clinical Transplantation of Cord Blood Cells

As part of a national multi-institutional study evaluating the harvesting, transport and numerical content of human hematopoietic progenitors in over 100 cord blood collections, and the cryopreservation and successful thawing of these cells, investigators in the author's laboratory had estimated that there are enough progenitor cells in a single cord blood collection for clinical transplantation and hematopoietic reconstitution.[9] These studies broadened into a wider national multi-institutional and international study coordinated in major part at Indiana University, where cord blood from an infant was transplanted into an HLA-matched sibling patient with Fanconi anemia.[12] Prenatal identification of potential donors for umbilical cord blood transplantation for patients with Fanconi anemia was available,[13] as was prenatal HLA typing.[14] Complete engraftment of the myeloid system with donor cells was evident from cytogenetics, ABO grouping, study of DNA polymorphism and normal cellular resistance to the cytotoxic agents that reveal the fragility of Fanconi anemia cells. The patient's blood contained residual host lymphocytes exhibiting chromosome damage, but after 1 year the lymphoid system was ≥98% of donor origin. This patient is now more than 6 years from umbilical cord blood transplant and is healthy and hematologically normal. Three other patients with

Fanconi anemia have been transplanted with HLA-matched sibling cord blood cells. These umbilical cord blood cells were assayed for progenitors and frozen at Indiana University, and hand-delivered to the transplant centers (Paris and Cincinnati).[15,16] Two of these three latter transplants were successful, and these patients are hematologically normal 3 and 4 years after transplant. The first cord blood transplant done with a truly myeloablative conditioning regimen was for a child with juvenile chronic myelogenous leukemia (CML).[17] Donor cell engraftment was documented in the patient's peripheral blood and bone marrow by cytogenetic analysis, restriction fragment length polymorphism and polymerase chain reaction by day 21 after transplant of HLA-matched sibling cord blood. The donor origin of lymphoid and myeloid lineage cells was confirmed. Recurrent disease was demonstrated histologically on day 225. The patient was subsequently transplanted with bone marrow from the donor of the cord blood. At the time of writing, there have been 50 transplants performed in children using HLA-matched sibling cord blood including Fanconi anemia, juvenile CML, Ph+CML, Ph+ acute lymphocytic leukemia, AUL, neuroblastoma, Wiscott-Aldrich syndrome, aplastic anemia and an X-linked lymphoproliferative disorder. There are reports in the literature for only a limited number of these transplants,[14-19] but it is interesting that the successful engraftment of a patient with an X-linked lymphoproliferative disorder[19] is the first reported success of hematopoietic transplantation in this disease. Three previous transplants with bone marrow as a source of stem cells were not successful in this disease.

There have also been a number of partially HLA-matched sibling cord blood transplants done in children. The only one reported in the literature is a two-antigen mismatch (one antigen mismatch in each direction) for ALL.[20] At least five three-antigen (1 haplotype) mismatched sibling cord blood transplants have been performed, but detailed information on these transplants is not yet available. Of great potential importance is the fact that sibling cord blood transplants performed so far have been associated with low to nondetectable levels of graft-vs-host disease (GVHD). Bone marrow transplants into children are believed to be associated with less GVHD than such transplants into adults. Thus, determination of whether cord blood transplants are truly associated with less GVHD than found with bone marrow awaits cord blood transplants in adults. The results thus far in children, however, are very encouraging.

Cord Blood Transplantation in Adults

A critical question that needed to be addressed is whether single collections of cord blood also contained sufficient numbers of immature cells to engraft the hematopoietic system of adults. When collections of bone marrow cells are made for autologous or allogeneic transplantation, it is usual to collect as many cells as possible. In contrast, what is collected from the cord blood is limited by what is present. Collection of an individual's cord blood is a one-time-only possibility.

The original calculations of MPCs in cord blood[9] were estimated by using either recombinant human GM-CSF or medium conditioned by the urinary bladder carcinoma cell line 5637 (5637 CM, a source of GM-CSF, other CSFs and interleukins) to stimulate colony formation of CFU-GM. Erythropoietin (EPO) plus either 5637 CM or IL-3 was used to stimulate colony formation of CFU-GEMM. EPO, with or without 5637 CM or IL-3, was used to stimulate colony formation of BFU-E. It is now known that there are a number of other cytokines that either directly or indirectly stimulate or enhance colony formation of MPCs and that these effects are synergistic, which suggests that the number of MPCs in cord blood collections was most likely underestimated. One of the newly identified growth factors is the potent costimulating cytokine, steel factor (SLF), which has also been termed mast cell growth factor, stem cell factor, and kit ligand.[21] Using SLF in combination with CSFs, the numbers of MPCs in cord blood were re-evaluated.[10] SLF plus GM-CSF allowed the detection of 8- to 11-fold more CFU-GM than was found when GM-CSF or 5637 CM was used as the stimulus. When SLF was added to EPO plus IL-3, 15-fold more CFU-GEMM were detected than when cells were stimulated with EPO plus either IL-3 or 5637 CM. Since SLF is an early-acting cytokine, it is likely that its use allows detection of early subpopulations of MPCs. Bone marrow CFU-GM and CFU-GEMM detection was also enhanced; however, the effect was not as great as that seen with cord blood. Recalculation based on this information suggests that, in all likelihood, there would have been enough stem and progenitor cells in a single collection of cord blood to repopulate the hematopoietic system of an adult.[10] Cord blood cells can grow for prolonged periods in long-term cultures.[22] Using long-term culture assays, other investigators have also suggested that single collections of cord blood will repopulate hematopoiesis in adults.[23,24] It is not only the quantity of progenitor cells that will dictate the engraftment potential of cells. The quality of these cells is also important, and this includes the proliferative and self-renewal capacities of the more immature cells. The proliferative capacity of early cord blood cells is extensive.[25-27]

In-Vitro Expansion of Progenitor Cells

Further information suggesting a more immature profile of early cells in cord blood vs bone marrow is based on the comparative replating capacity of CFU-GEMM and high proliferative potential colony-forming cells (HPP-CFC) in cord blood and bone marrow.[25-27] Replating capability is used as an estimate of the self-renewal capacity of early cells. Self-renewal, the ability of a stem cell to duplicate itself, is extremely important in the maintenance of blood cell production, but it is a poorly understood event.[8]

Assuming that some cord blood collections may not contain enough progenitor cells to ensure engraftment in an adult, or that one might want to use the cells from one cord blood collection for more than one recipient, the ability to expand numbers of stem and progenitor cells in vitro would be a tremendous advancement. Unfortunately, there is no assay yet available to characterize and quantitate the human marrow repopulating cells, although such assays are apparently available for murine cells.[28] Efforts to expand cells have been successful but have relied for the most part on quantitation of progenitor cells.[10,23,24] More recently, bioreactors have been suggested as a means for large-scale expansion of cells.[29] Large-scale expansion of early bone marrow cells has been accomplished in continuous perfusion cultures.[30] Whether these expansions truly reflect expansion or even maintenance of marrow repopulating cells is still unknown. It is possible that progenitor values will reflect the levels of repopulating cells, but extreme caution is still warranted in using such a correlation.

Cord Blood Banks

The use of umbilical cord blood cells has been shown to be efficacious in the setting of HLA-matched siblings for tranplantation in children. Analysis of the cellular contents of single cord blood collections suggests that such cells may also be efficacious in adults. It is of interest that little GVHD has been noted in the recipients of HLA-matched sibling cord blood. This may reflect the immature nature of cord blood cells. Still to be defined is the broadness of applicability of cord blood as a source of transplantable cells in the context of partially mismatched cells, cells from unrelated donors and transplants with adults as recipients. Cord blood banks are imperative for the answers to these questions and are being developed. A number of considerations have been covered in detail with regards to cord blood banks.[31] Presently, the New York Blood Center is funded by a National Institutes of Health grant to determine the feasibility of and problems associated with collection, typing, assessment and storage of a large number of cord and placental blood samples. In addition, a private company, Biocyte Corporation (Stamford, CT), is also evaluating these problems. Cord blood banks could potentially allow access to stored samples of HLA types not presently available through bone marrow registries, especially for minority groups. The only perfectly matched set of cells is one's own. The author envisions a time when the cord blood of all newborns will be collected and stored for their own future use, and cord blood banks will be available with HLA-typed cells for allogeneic transplantation to related and unrelated recipients. Cord blood banks should interrelate well with the National Marrow Donor Program and the International Marrow Registry.

For those interested in cord blood transplantation, there are a number of logistical considerations. It was found early on that even the simplest separation of cells led to unacceptable losses in progenitor cell numbers in cord blood and that attempts to wash cryopreserved cord blood cells after thawing also led to unacceptable losses of cells.[9,15] On the basis of these considerations, the first five cord blood transplants[14-17] and many of the subsequent cord blood transplants were done without any separation of cells (no removal of red cells, platelets or granulocytes) and without washing of cells after thawing. Some investigators have reported reasonable yields of progenitor cells after simple fractionation of the cells,[32] but it is important to be aware that large losses can occur upon cell separation. Unless expansion of early cells becomes a reality, one cannot get more of these cells. It is not known how few cord blood cells can be used for successful engraftment, and one would want to make sure that as many cells as possible are available for transplantation purposes. In this context, collection of as many cells as possible from the cord and placenta becomes important.[11] Theoretically, once cells are frozen, they can be retrieved in viable form after an "indefinite" period of time in a frozen state. Cord blood progenitor cells have been frozen and retrieved in viable form after 6 years,[10] and human marrow cyropreserved for up to 11 years has been found to be capable of engraftment.[33] Thus, it seems reasonable to assume that cord blood banking is a realistic endeavor.

The complete context within which cord blood can and will be used is open to investigation. In-utero transplantation has been studied in higher animals, including sheep and monkey models.[34,35] The idea is to utilize fetal tolerance by injecting cells in-utero at early gestation periods. Cord blood might be useful in this context; fetal liver cells have already been used.[36] Cord blood cells are easily transduced with genes present in retroviral vectors,[37,38] and cord blood cells may be an excellent vehicle for such vectors for correction of metabolic disorders and other genetic diseases. In fact, transduction of cord blood with genes has already been used in an autologous situation shortly after birth. Obviously, much remains to be learned. Further research into characterization of the earliest cells in cord blood is needed. Are there cells present in cord blood that can give rise to both the hematopoietic microenvironment and hematopoietic stem cells? Research is also needed on the expansion of these cells and the immunologic reactivity inherent in cells within cord blood collections.

Acknowledgments

I thank Rebecca Miller for typing this manuscript, and all the collaborators with whom I am listed as author or co-author on the papers in the reference section, for their important contributions to the work described.

References

1. Broxmeyer HE, Williams DE. The production of myeloid blood cells and their regulation during health and disease. CRC Crit Rev Oncol/Hematol 1988;8:173-226.

2. Williams DE, Lu L, Broxmeyer HE. Characterization of hematopoietic stem and progenitor cells. Surv Immunol Rev 1987;6:294-304.
3. Thomas ED. Frontiers in bone marrow transplantation. Blood Cells 1991;17:259-67.
4. Lowry RA, Tabbara IA. Peripheral hematopoietic stem cell transplantation: Current concepts. Exp Hematol 1992; 20:937-42.
5. Tavassoli M. Embryonic and fetal hematopoiesis: An overview. Blood Cells 1991;17:269-81.
6. Touraine JL, Roncarolo MG, Royo C, Touraine F. Fetal tissue transplantation, bone marrow transplantation and prospective gene therapy in severe immunodeficiencies and enzyme deficiencies. Thymus 1987;10:75-87.
7. Gale RP. Fetal liver transplants. Bone Marrow Transplant 1992;9 (Suppl 1):118-20.
8. Broxmeyer HE. Self-renewal and migration of stem cells during embryonic and fetal hematopoiesis: Important, but poorly understood events. Blood Cells 1991;17:282-6.
9. Broxmeyer HD, Douglas GW, Hangoc G, et al. Human umbilical cord blood as a potential source of transplantable hematopoietic stem/progenitor cells. Proc Natl Acad Sci USA 1989;86:3828-32.
10. Broxmeyer HE, Hangoc G, Cooper S, et al. Growth characteristics and expansion of human umbilical cord blood and estimation of its potential for transplantation of adults. Proc Natl Acad Sci USA 1992;89:4109-13.
11. Wagner JE, Broxmeyer HE, Cooper S. Umbilical cord and placental blood hematopoietic stem cells: collection, cryopreservation, and storage. J Hematother 1992;1:167-73.
12. Gluckman E, Broxmeyer HE, Auerbach AD, et al. Hematopoietic reconstitution in a patient with Fanconi's anemia by means of umbilical-cord blood from an HLA-identical sibling. N Engl J Med 1989;321:1174-8.
13. Auerbach AD, Liu Q, Ghosh R, et al. Prenatal identification of potential donors for umbilical cord blood transplantation for Fanconi anemia. Transfusion 1990;30:682-7.
14. Pollack MS, Auerbach AD, Broxmeyer HE, et al. DNA amplification for DQ typing as an adjunct to serological prenatal HLA typing for the identification of potential donors for umbilical cord blood transplantation. Hum Immunol 1991;30:45-9.

15. Broxmeyer HE, Kurtzberg J, Gluckman E, et al. Umbilical cord blood hematopoietic stem and repopulating cells in human clinical transplantation. Blood Cells 1991;17:313-29.
16. Kohli-Kumar M, Shahidi NT, Broxmeyer HE, et al. Haematopoietic stem/progenitor cell transplant in Fanconi anemia using HLA-matched sibling umbilical cord blood cells. Br J Haematol 1993;85:419-22.
17. Wagner JE, Broxmeyer HE, Byrd RL, et al. Transplantation of umbilical cord blood after myeloblative therapy: Analysis of engraftment. Blood 1992;79:1874-81.
18. Broxmeyer HE, Hangoc G, Cooper S. Clinical and biological aspects of human umbilical cord blood as a source of transplantable hematopoietic stem and progenitor cells. Bone Marrow Transplant 1992;9(Suppl 1):7-10.
19. Vowels MR, Tang RLP, Bendoukas V, et al. Correction of X-linked lymphoproliferative disease by cord blood transplantation. N Engl J Med 1994;20:249-55.
20. Vilmer E, Broyart A, Lescoeur B, et al. HLA-mismatched cord blood transplantation in a patient with advanced leukemia. Transplantation 1992;53:1155-7.
21. Broxmeyer HE, Maze R, Miyazawa K, et al. The kit receptor and its ligand, steel factor, as regulators of hemopoiesis. Cancer Cells 1991;3:480-7.
22. Smith S, Broxmeyer HE. The influence of oxygen tension on the long term growth in vitro of haematopoietic progenitor cells from human cord blood. Br J Haematol 1986;53:29-34.
23. Hows JM, Bradley BA, Marsh JCW, et al. Growth of human umbilical-cord blood in long term haematopoietic cultures. Lancet 1992;340:73-6.
24. Cardoso AA, Li ML, Hatzfeld A, et al. Release from quiescence of CD34+CD38- human umbilical cord blood cells reveals their potentiality to engraft adults. Proc Natl Acad Sci USA 1993; 90:8707-11.
25. Carow CE, Hangoc G, Cooper SH, et al. Mast cell growth factor (c-kit ligand) supports the growth of human multipotential (CFU-GEMM) progenitor cells with a high replating potential. Blood 1991;78:2216-21.
26. Carow CE, Hangoc G, Broxmeyer HE. Human multipotential progenitor cells (CFU-GEMM) have extensive replating capacity for secondary CFU-GEMM: An effect enhanced by cord blood plasma. Blood 1993;81:942-9.

27. Lu L, Xiao M, Shen RN, et al. Enrichment, characterization and responsiveness of single primitive CD34^{+++} human umbilical cord blood hematopoietic progenitors with high proliferative and replating potential. Blood 1993;81:41-8.
28. Harrison DE, Jordan CT, Zhong RK, Astle CM. Primitive hemopoietic stem cells: Direct assay of most productive populations by competitive repopulation with simple binomial, correlation and covariance calculations. Exp Hematol 1993;21:206-19.
29. Edgington SM. New horizons for stem cell bioreactors. Biotechnology 1992;10:1099-106.
30. Koller MR, Emerson SG, Palsson BO. Large-scale expansion of human stem and progenitor cells in continuous perfusion cultures. Blood 1993;82:378-84.
31. Rubinstein P, Rosenfeld RE, Adamson JW, Stevens CE. Stored placental blood for unrelated bone marrow reconstitution. Blood 1993;81:1679-90.
32. Newton I, Charbord P, School JP, Herve P. Toward cord blood banking: density-separation and cryopreservation of cord blood progenitors. Exp Hematol 1993;21:671-4.
33. Aird W, Labopin M, Gorin NC, Antin JH. Long-term cyropreservation of human stem cells. Bone Marrow Transplant 1992;9:487-90.
34. Flake AW, Harrison MR, Zanjani ED. In utero stem cell transplantation. Exp Hematol 1991;19:1061-4.
35. Zanjani ED, Ascensao JL, Flake AW, et al. The fetus as an optimal donor and recipient of hemopoietic stem cells. Bone Marrow Transplant 1992;10(Suppl 1):107-14.
36. Flake AW, Harrison MR, Adzick NS, Zanjani ED. Transplantation of fetal hematopoietic stem cells in utero: The creation of hematopoietic chimeras. Science 1986;233:776-8.
37. Moritz T, Keller DC, Williams DA. Human cord blood cells as targets for gene transfer: potential use in genetic therapies of severe combined immunodeficiency disease. J Exp Med 1993;178:529-36.
38. Lu L, Xiao M, Clapp DW, Li ZH, Broxmeyer HE. High efficiency retroviral mediated gene transduction into single isolated immature and replatable CD34^{+++} hematopoietic stem/progenitor cells from human umbilical cord blood. J Exp Med 1993;178:2089-96.

In: Lasky L and Warkentin P, eds. *Marrow and Stem Cell
Processing for Transplantation*
Bethesda, MD: American Association of Blood Banks, 1995

12

Ex-Vivo Expansion of CD34⁺ Progenitor Cells

Shelly Heimfeld, PhD; Ruigao Fei, MD; Zhenna Tsui, BA; Barbra
Fogarty, BA; Penny Thompson, BA; and Ronald J. Berenson, MD

THE ABILITY TO EXPAND PROGENITOR CELLS ex-vivo has broad potential for therapeutic benefit. We have focused on defining conditions that make expansion clinically practical. The CEPRATE® stem cell selection system has been used to isolate large numbers of CD34⁺ progenitor cells from human bone marrow for growth in suspension culture with recombinant cytokines. The cultured cells were analyzed for overall expansion (defined as fold-increase over the inoculated value) in total cell numbers, total CD34⁺ cells, and colony-forming activity. Our results indicate that CD34 enrichment enhances expansion 10-fold as compared with unseparated marrow. Addition of 5% human plasma augments growth 5- to 20-fold. Optimal expansion requires combinations of at least four cytokines. Using SCF+ IL-1+ IL-3+ IL-6 results in a 30- to 50-fold-increase in progenitor cells by 7-14 days of culture. With no media exchange, optimal expansion occurs at starting cell densities of $<1 \times 10^5$ cells/mL. Frequent media replacement allows >10-fold expansion at plating densities of $1-4 \times 10^6$ CD34⁺ cells/mL. These results indicate that large quantities of CD34⁺ progenitor cells can be isolated and expanded in a clinically practical fashion ex vivo for subsequent transplantation.

The bone marrow is the primary site of hematopoiesis in adult vertebrates, and it contains the precursor cells that ultimately give rise to all the various blood cells. The earliest progenitors

Shelly Heimfeld, PhD, Director of Biological Research; Ruigao Fei, MD, Scientist; Zhenna Tsui, BA, Research Associate; Barbra Fogarty, BA, Research Associate; Penny Thompson, BA, Research Associate; and Ronald J. Berenson, MD, Executive Vice President, Chief Medical and Scientific Officer; CellPro, Inc, Bothell, Washington have been termed stem cells. They are defined by their capacity for self-renewal and their ability to differentiate into multiple cell types. Self-renewal can be roughly defined as proliferation without loss of further proliferative or differentiation potential. The property of self-renewal is the hallmark of stem cells and distinguishes them from all the other cells in the marrow. It is generally believed that stem cells first give rise to more restricted precursor cells; these in turn generate unipotent progenitors through a poorly understood series of differentiation steps. These lineage-committed cells then mature into various specialized end cells (Fig 12-1). Most mature blood cells have a limited life span of a few days to several weeks. Thus, to maintain the steady-state levels found in normal individuals, these mature cellular elements must be continuously produced.

Integral to the hierarchy of hematopoietic stem cells and progenitors are control mechanisms that influence these precursors to modulate their growth and output of differentiated cells. This regulatory machinery can be viewed as an intricate network that permits communication of hematopoietic cells among themselves, with various bone marrow stromal elements and with the extracellular matrix. It is these layers of communication that form the positive and negative feedback loops that give the hematopoietic system its remarkable homeostatic and renewal properties. Thus, following high-dose myeloablative therapy,

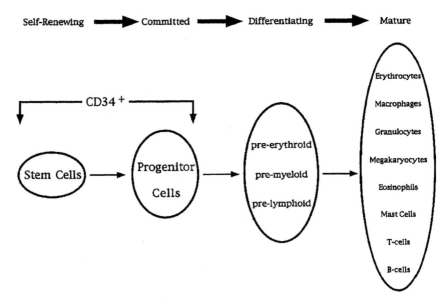

Figure 12-1. Model of hematopoietic development.

infusion of a relatively small number of stem and progenitor cells can completely regenerate the lymphoid and myeloid compartments of the bone marrow in transplant patients.

Use of Growth-Factor-Dependent Culture Systems

Culture systems have been developed that allow early hematopoietic cells to proliferate and differentiate in an ex-vivo environment. These systems can be classified into two distinct categories: 1) bone marrow cultures, in which a mix of accessory cells supports the growth of the precursor populations[1,2] and 2) growth-factor-dependent cultures in which the progenitors grow in media supplemented with various cytokines[3] This chapter discusses systems of the second type.

In the absence of direct accessory cell support, stem and progenitor cell proliferation is dependent on a set of glycoproteins collectively termed growth factors. Many of these factors have now been cloned and purified to homogeneity (Table 12-1). Specific details as to the cellular sources for these factors, the amounts of factors found in different tissues and factor modula-

Table 12-1. Hematopoietic Growth Factors*

Factor	Abbreviation	Other Synonyms
Erythropoietin	EPO	—
Macrophage colony-stimulating factor	M-CSF	CSF-1
Granulocyte colony-stimulating factor	G-CSF	Pluripoietin, CSF-β
Granulocyte macrophage colony-stimulating factor	GM-CSF	Pluripoietin-alpha
Interleukin-1	IL-1	Hemopoietin-1
Interleukin-2	IL-2	TCGF
Interleukin-3	IL-3	Multi-CSF, HCGF
Interleukin-4	IL-4	BCGF
Interleukin-6	IL-6	BSF-2, IFN-β2
Stem cell factor	SCF	SF, KL, MCGF

* The factors listed here represent only a partial catalog of previously characterized cytokines that have been shown to exert some influence on hematopoiesis in culture.

tion in response to changing demands have been reviewed elsewhere.[4] Unique cell surface receptors have been found for many of these factors. Many progenitor cells can simultaneously express receptors for more than one factor and, therefore, can proliferate in response to multiple factors. It is also important to emphasize that culture conditions have not yet been defined that can match the efficiency of stem cell self-renewal that occurs during ontogeny or during hematopoietic recovery following myeloablative therapy. Identification of new factors that may mediate this process thus continues to pose a major challenge to many basic and applied studies, including those focused on leukemogenesis, cancer treatment and gene therapy.

Ex-Vivo Expansion of Progenitor Cells

The ex-vivo proliferation of hematopoietic progenitor cells has the potential to provide several important clinical benefits. It could lead to a reduction in bone marrow or apheresis harvest requirements, since a smaller number of cells could be expanded to support transplantation after myelosuppressive therapy. By virtue of activating the progenitor cells and enhancing certain stages of differentiation, expansion could potentially lead to more rapid engraftment. Ex-vivo expansion could be used to support dose-escalation of chemotherapy, which might lead to better cure rates. In the same vein, expanded cells might be purged of contaminating tumor cells during the culture period, thereby reducing the incidence of relapse. Finally, ex-vivo culture is a critical element in most current gene therapy protocols, and improved expansion methods might enhance this emerging area of clinical research.

The purpose of the experiments reported here was to determine the conditions necessary to make ex-vivo expansion practical in the clinical setting. Toward this goal, it is critical that the stem and progenitor cells first be enriched and concentrated, primarily to reduce the total number of cells and thus the volume of material to be cultured, but also to remove potentially inhibitory cells that can interfere with the expansion.

A New System

Hematopoietic progenitor and stem cells express a unique antigen, designated CD34, that is not found on mature blood cells or on most types of malignant cells.[5] CellPro, Inc, (Bothell, WA) has designed a unique avidin-biotin immunoadsorption system (CEPRATE® SC) for clinical-scale purification of CD34⁺ cells. The basic components of the CEPRATE® SC system include a biotin-conjugated CD34 monoclonal antibody, which is used specifically to mark the stem and progenitor cells in bone marrow, and a column that contains avidin-coated beads. When antibody-labeled cells flow through the column, the strong affinity between biotin and avidin results in specific capture of the stem cells, while the unwanted (unlabeled) cells continue and exit the column. The purified stem cells are then released from the column by gentle agitation and washing, and are collected for further processing or cryopreservation. This system has now been used in a wide variety of clinical settings, and the results indicate that enriched CD34⁺ bone marrow cells can engraft and reconstitute patients after high-dose myeloablative chemotherapy.[6-9] It is these enriched CD34⁺ cells that have been used as the starting material for our ex-vivo expansion experiments.

Several variables were evaluated to determine optimal expansion conditions for CD34⁺ selected cells. The results from those experiments indicate several facts. 1) Expansion of enriched CD34⁺ cells is 5- to 20-fold greater than that seen with whole bone marrow. 2) Minimal growth is obtained when only a single cytokine is used, while two-, three- or four-factor combinations result in the production of increasing amounts of progenitor cells and total cells in the cultures. The best combinations include stem cell factor and interleukins 1, 3 and 6. 3) Plating cell density has a major influence on the expansion of CD34⁺ cells. Densities below 10^4 cells/mL give significant expansion, while above 10^6 cells/mL growth is inhibited. 4) Supplementing "serum-free" basal medium with 5-10% autologous plasma or serum enhances expansion several-fold. Optimal culture time was also investigated. Total cell numbers continue to increase for several weeks during culture; however, progenitor cell numbers appear to peak at 7-11 days[10,11] (also: Heimfeld S, et al, unpublished observations).

Summary

The ability to expand progenitor cells ex-vivo has broad potential for therapeutic benefit. Investigators are currently defining conditions that make expansion clinically practical. The CEPRATE®

stem cell selection system has been used to isolate large numbers of CD34$^+$ progenitor cells from human bone marrow for growth in suspension culture with recombinant cytokines. The cultured cells were analyzed for overall expansion (defined as fold-increase over the inoculated value) in total cell numbers, total CD34$^+$ cells and colony-forming activity. Results indicate that CD34 enrichment enhances expansion >10-fold as compared with unseparated marrow. Addition of 5% human plasma augments growth 5- to 20-fold. Optimal expansion requires combinations of at least four cytokines. Using stem cell factor with interleukins 1, 3 and 6 results in a 30- to 50-fold increase in progenitor cells by 7-14 days of culture. With no media exchange, optimal expansion occurs at starting cell densities of <1 × 10^5 cells/mL. Frequent media replacment allows >10-fold expansion at plating densities of 1-4 × 10^6 CD34$^+$ cells/mL. These results indicate that large quantities of CD34$^+$ progenitor cells can be isolated and expanded in a clinically practical fashion ex vivo for subsequent transplantation.

With this methodology, progenitor cell growth can be reproducibly accomplished and easily moved up to a therapeutic scale. Clinical trials testing the safety and efficacy of ex-vivo expanded cells are expected to begin in the near future.

References

1. Barnett MJ, Eaves CJ, Phillips GL, et al. Successful autografting in chronic myeloid leukemia after maintenance of marrow in culture. Bone Marrow Transplant 1989;4:345-51.
2. Chang J, Morgenstern GR, Coutinho LH, et al. The use of bone marrow cells grown in long-term culture for autologous bone marrow transplantation in acute myeloid leukemia: An update. Bone Marrow Transplant 1989;4:5-9.
3. Moore MAS. Clinical implications of positive and negative hematopoietic stem cell regulators. Blood 1991;78:1-11.
4. Metcalf D. Hematopoietic regulators: Redundancy or subtlety? Blood 1993;82:3515-23.
5. Civin CI, Gore SD. Antigenic analysis of hematopoiesis: A review. J Hematother 1993;2:137-44.
6. Berenson RJ, Bensinger WI, Andrews RG, et al. Hematopoietic stem cell transplants. In: Gale RP, Golde DW, eds. Recent advances in leukemia and lymphoma. New York: Alan R. Liss, 1987:527-33.

7. Berenson RJ, Bensinger WI, Kalamasz D, et al. Avidin-biotin immunoadsorption: A technique to purify cells and its potential applications. In: Gale RP, Champlin R, eds. Progress in bone marrow transplantation. New York: Alan R. Liss, 1987:423-8.

8. Shpall EJ, Stemmer SM, Johnston CF, et al. Purging of autologous bone marrow for transplantation: The protection and selection of the hematopoietic progenitor cell. J Hematother 1992;1:45-54.

9. Shpall EJ, Jones RB, Bearman SI, et al. Transplantation of enriched CD34-positive autologous marrow into breast cancer patients following high-dose chemotherapy: Influence of CD34-positive peripheral blood progenitors and growth factors on engraftment. J Clin Oncol 1994;12:28-36.

10. Haylock DN, To LB, Dowse TL, et al. Ex vivo expansion and maturation of peripheral blood CD34+ cells into the myeloid lineage. Blood 1992;80:1405-12.

11. Brugger W, Möcklin W, Heimfeld S, et al. Ex vivo expansion of enriched peripheral blood CD34+ progenitor cells by stem cell factor, interleukin-1β (IL-1β), IL-6, IL-3, interferon-γ, and erythropoietin. Blood 1993;81:2579-84.

In: Lasky L and Warkentin P, eds. *Marrow and Stem Cell Processing for Transplantation*
Bethesda, MD: American Association of Blood Banks, 1995

13

Isolation of Human Hematopoietic Stem Cells

Irwin D. Bernstein, MD; Robert G. Andrews, MD; and Scott Rowley, MD

HEMATOPOIESIS ENTAILS CONTROLLING the proliferation and differentiation of hematopoietic cells and providing for renewal of the primitive stem cells, for maturation of these cells to achieve adequate numbers of circulating mature blood cells and for expansion of specific cell lineages in response to disease states such as infection or blood loss. Blood cells arise from totipotential stem cells.[1] These rare, quiescent cells compose a distinct subpopulation of the hematopoietic cells with proliferative capacity. Daughter cells, further along the maturational pathways, are thought to be more limited in self-renewal and differentiative potential and are more likely to be actively proliferative, or in cell cycle, at any given time.[2]

Inherent to this stem cell model is the existence of a hierarchical heterogeneity of hematopoietic progenitors. The more mature hematopoietic progenitor cells may be cloned in vitro, giving rise to colonies containing cells of single or multiple lineages [eg, colony-forming units–granulocyte/macrophage (CFU-GM), burst-forming units–erythroid (BFU-E) and colony-forming units–granulocyte/erythroid/megakaryocyte/macrophage (CFU-GEMM)] that presumably reflect the maturational potential of the

Irwin D. Bernstein, MD, Member, Fred Hutchinson Cancer Research Center, and Professor of Pediatrics, University of Washington; Robert G. Andrews, MD, Associate Member, Fred Hutchinson Cancer Research Center, and Associate Professor of Pediatrics, University of Washington; and Scott Rowley, MD, Assistant Member, Fred Hutchinson Cancer Research Center, Seattle, Washington
(This work was supported in part by NIH grants and contracts CA39492 and N01-AI-85003.)

individual progenitor cell.[3-10] This terminology unfortunately leads to viewing hematopoiesis as occurring in discrete stages. Rather, hematopoietic development is a continuum from the earliest stem cell to late progenitor cell and, ultimately, to mature blood cell. Hence, a class of progenitor cells defined in-vitro by certain characteristics may still be markedly heterogeneous. The relative contributions of cells with defined in-vitro potentials to hematologic recovery after marrow transplantation have not been determined in human transplantation, as infusion of purified populations highly enriched for or depleted of hematopoietic progenitor cells of various maturational stages has not been performed. After transplantation of marrow into recipients treated with myeloablative therapy, cells at all stages of maturation presumably contribute to the hematologic recovery, although engraftment and survival of adequate numbers of pluripotent stem cells are thought to be necessary for sustained production of donor-derived cells.[11] Whether the proportion of more mature to primitive hematopoietic progenitor cells explains the different kinetics of hematologic recovery frequently observed when marrow- and blood-derived cells are infused is not known. The infusion of inadequate numbers of the appropriate cell type may lead to nonengraftment or delayed graft failure.[11]

During the past decade, the possibility of identifying and isolating putative human hematopoietic stem cells from bone marrow, peripheral blood or umbilical cord blood has become a reality. As a consequence of these recent advances, this book is focused to a great extent on methods for isolating and storing these cells, removing potentially contaminating tumor cells and expanding these populations in vitro for subsequent use in vivo. This chapter discusses the background data providing evidence that the CD34 antigen is expressed by pluripotent hematopoietic stem cells capable of reconstituting hematopoiesis in patients following myeloablative therapy. First, evidence is reviewed from nonhuman primate and human studies demonstrating that CD34+ cells, but not CD34− cells, can reconstitute the multiple hematopoietic lineages. Second, data are presented showing that the subpopulation of CD34+ cells that does not express antigens associated with commitment to individual hematopoietic lineages (CD34+Lin−), a population less mature than the CD34+Lin+ colony-forming cell population, is responsible for this multi-lineage engraftment. Third, in-vitro conditions required for detecting and growing these immature precursor populations are discussed.

Evidence That the CD34+ Hematopoietic Precursors Contain the Pluripotent Hematopoietic Stem Cell

The CD34 antigen is a 115-kD glycoprotein of unknown function that is present on 2-4% of bone marrow cells.[12-17] The CD34+ marrow cell population contains the least mature myeloid and lymphoid cells (as determined by morphology),[12,13] the vast majority of hematopoietic myeloid colony-forming cells[12-17] and less mature cells that are the precursors of the colony-forming cells.[15] Xenogeneic models have been used to demonstrate the derivation of T- and B-lymphoid cells from CD34+ precursor cells.[18-21] Recent studies have provided in-vivo evidence arguing that pluripotent stem cells responsible for long-term maintenance of all of the hematopoietic lineages after transplantation are indeed within the CD34+ population.[22-24]

Preclinical Studies

Initial evidence that the CD34+ marrow cell population was capable of establishing hematopoiesis following myeloablative treatment came from studies of nonhuman primates. This was possible as one CD34 antibody, 12.8, was found to detect an epitope present on nonhuman primate marrow cells. According to Berenson et al.,[22] it was possible to demonstrate that partially purified autologous CD34+ marrow cells would reconstitute hematopoiesis in baboons following a dose of total-body irradiation thought to be myeloablative. The cells were partially purified using a solid-phase immunoadsorption chromatography method in which 12.8 antibody-coated cells were labeled with a biotinylated antimouse immunoglobulin antibody, adsorbed to avidin-coated beads in a column and then eluted by agitation of the beads. Three animals received $4.2 \pm 0.2 \times 10^6$ cells per kilogram of partially purified autologous marrow cells that were 65-81% CD34+. Two additional animals received cells that were further purified by fluorescence-activated cell sorting (FACS) (3.2 and 3.9×10^6 per kg), and were 85% and 91% CD34+. Animals that received column-enriched cells all engrafted and displayed hyperplastic marrow with evidence of engraftment of each of the myeloid lineages. These animals, however, died of a presumed posttransplant viral syndrome. It is important to note that the two baboons that received the column- and FACS-purified cells experienced long-term engraftment (more than 2 and 4 years).

Control animals that received unseparated autologous marrow ($2.1 \pm 0.1 \times 10^8$ cells per kg) engrafted at the same rate as those receiving enriched CD34+ cells. In contrast, of two animals that received marrow depleted of CD34+ cells ($2.3 \pm 0.7 \times 10^8$ cells per kg), one died with an aplastic marrow and the other demonstrated a partial and substantially delayed reconstitution.

In the absence of a marker to distinguish infused autologous cells from residual host cells that may have escaped the myeloablative treatment, the preceding experiments only demonstrated the ability of CD34+ cells to provide an early wave of rapid engraftment, but they did not prove that the long-term hematopoietic activity observed in the two long-term survivors was due to the infused cells. To answer this question, pairs of sex-mismatched sibling baboons that were matched on the basis of nonreactivity in mixed leukocyte culture were identified.[24] This allowed transplantation of allogeneic CD34+ marrow cells in which the sex chromosomes served as markers for donor and host cells. In these studies, the CD34+ cells were further purified and depleted of cells displaying antigens associated with T and B lymphocytes and mature myeloid cells. Thus, these cells, which in all cases were greater than 95% CD34+, were also depleted of mature and immature lymphocytes. In all animals, the initial hematopoietic reconstitution was from infused donor cells, which confirms observations from the autologous transplant studies. In three successful transplants in which long-term survival was obtained, it was possible to demonstrate that the myeloid and lymphoid lineages were derived from the infused donor cells, almost completely in two animals and partially in the third. These animals have maintained stable lymphohematopoietic chimerism in the absence of immunosuppression for more than 2 years, and a third has done so for more than 1 year. These experiments, therefore, proved that infused CD34+ cells could contribute to hematopoiesis in the long term. Moreover, their ability to give rise to cells in both the lymphoid and myeloid lineages over time strongly suggests that the cell responsible for this long-term multilineage activity is a pluripotent CD34+ cell.

Clinical Studies

In humans, CD34+ cells have been used as a source of stem cells when the separation of these cells from tumor cells may be beneficial. Evidence has indicated that selectively isolating CD34+ marrow cells by using an immunoadsorption column, as described above, may allow these cells to be separated from contaminating tumor cells that lack CD34 antigen expression. Infusions of column-enriched autologous CD34+ bone marrow cells ($2.4 \pm 1.5 \times 10^6$ cells per kg), which were 62-92% CD34+ led to the establishment of hematopoiesis after myeloablative therapy in patients with breast cancer and neuroblastoma.[23] As noted above, this type of experiment does not prove that long-term multilineage engraftment was derived from the infused cells, but it does demonstrate that engraftment can be achieved by infusion of these cells. Since that initial result, Shpall et al[25] have shown in studies of patients with breast cancer that column-enriched CD34+ cells derived from marrow and/or blood of patients pretreated with granulocyte colony-stimulating factor led to rapid engraftment after high-dose chemotherapy.

Other in-vivo experiments have indicated that the cell within the CD34+ population responsible for long-term hematopoiesis is a CD34+ cell less mature than the CD34+ colony-forming cell population detectable by its coexpression of the CD33 antigen. In-vitro studies had indicated that normal and malignant CD34+ progenitors are separable from one another on the basis of expression of CD33.[26,27] In the in-vivo studies of Robertson et al,[28] both the normal and the malignant colony-forming cells were depleted from the marrow by the use of CD33 antibodies as a method of purging leukemic stem cells while sparing marrow-repopulating hematopoietic stem cells. While there is no definitive evidence that this method decreases the risk of relapse following high-dose chemoradiotherapy followed by autologous marrow transplantation in the treatment of acute myelogenous leukemia (AML), the results of these studies do demonstrate that CD33− cells must be responsible for hematopoietic reconstitution. Since delayed engraftment was observed with these cells, these studies suggested that the initial wave of hematopoietic engraftment is due to the CD34+CD33+ cells, presumably the colony-forming cells, while long-term hematopoiesis is provided by the CD34+CD33− cells. Similarly, the cyclophosphamide derivative, 4-hydroperoxycyclophosphamide (4-HC) has been used to eliminate AML precursors while sparing the hematopoietic stem cell.[29,30] This treatment also eliminates colony-forming cells and spares stem cells that are capable of engraftment, albeit with delayed kinetics compared with untreated marrow or enriched CD34+ cells. Other studies using antibodies against antigens associated with T or B cells to purge acute lymphocytic leukemic cells from marrow prior to autologous infusion have demonstrated that these antigens are not expressed on the hematopoietic stem cell.[31-34]

Studies in fetal sheep have been reported to show that human CD34+Lin– HLA/DR^{low} cells can give rise to progeny of different lymphohematopoietic lineages.[21] Verfaillie and colleagues have reported that normal and chronic myelogenous leukemia (CML) precursors are separable in in-vitro assays based on expression of HLA-DR, with bcr/abl-negative precursors being CD34+HLA-DR–.[35] In the following sections, the in-vitro conditions required to detect these immature subsets of CD34+ cells are discussed.

In-Vitro Correlates and Conditions for Propagating CD34+ Cell Subsets

As noted above, CD34+ cells were initially shown to contain nearly all of the colony-forming cells present in the marrow.[12-17] Subsequent studies demonstrated the presence of less mature precursors in this population, including precursors of blast colony-forming cells and cells that would give rise to colony-forming cells in long-term culture.[15,36] These primitive precursor cells were further identified as CD34+, but lacking expression of the CD33 antigen, known to be present on virtually all CFU-GM and most of the less mature erythroid precursors, BFU-E.[36,37] As described in the section above, this CD34+CD33– population must contain the hematopoietic stem cell based on the in-vivo repopulating activity of enriched CD34+ cells as well as marrow depleted of CD33+ cells.

More recent studies have examined conditions for inducing the generation of colony-forming cells from these CD34+ populations depleted of lineage-committed (Lin+) colony-forming cells such as CFU-GM or BFU-E. For the most part, these cells have been isolated through the use of a variety of antibodies that detect differentiation antigens associated with hematopoietic cells committed to individual lineages, to remove mature colony-forming cells and allow only their precursors (Lin–) to remain.[38-40] Other studies have isolated populations of CD34+ cells with similar characteristics based on their lack of expression of HLA-DR or CD38.[41-45]

In initial studies, it was not possible to grow CD34+Lin– cells in culture in the absence of marrow stroma. However, with the discovery of the hematopoietic growth factor known as steel factor, (mast cell growth factor or stem cell factor), it was possible to generate multiple colony-forming cells from individual CD34+Lin– precursors when this factor was combined with one or more of the other known growth factors, eg, granulocyte colony-stimulating factor or interleukin-3 (IL-3).[38] Thus, a substantial synergism was seen when multiple growth factors were combined, including, in particular, steel factor. These studies, therefore, demonstrated requirements for the generation of colony-forming activity that were distinct for these cells, as the more mature colony-forming cells would proliferate in the presence of single growth factors.

The question remains as to whether these growth factor combinations that stimulate the growth of the CD34+Lin– cells also stimulate the growth of the most primitive pluripotent stem cell, a cell thought to be quiescent. We have tested this possibility by examining the influence of hematopoietic growth factors, including steel factor, on the generation of colony-forming cells from a primitive and presumably quiescent population of CD34+Lin– cells selected on the basis of resistance to treatment with 4-HC.[40] This approach was used, because treatment of marrow with this drug (used to purge AML cells from marrow prior to autologous infusion) eliminates the colony-forming cells but spares hematopoietic stem cells capable of reconstituting hematopoiesis after myeloablative therapy. The observed tempo of engraftment following infusion of these cells is, however, slower than that observed with untreated marrow, presumably as a result of the absence of the colony-forming cell population, as in the case of marrow depleted of CD33-bearing cells.

The next question is whether the culture conditions required to stimulate the generation of colony-forming cells from CD34+Lin– cells from 4-HC-treated marrow were the same as or different from those required to stimulate their generation from untreated CD34+Lin– marrow cells. As noted above, steel factor, in combination with other hematopoietic growth factors including IL-1, IL-3, IL-6, GM-CSF or G-CSF caused untreated, but not 4-HC-treated, CD34+Lin– cells to form colony-forming cells.[40] It was, however, possible to generate colony-forming progeny from CD34+Lin– cells treated with 60 µg/mL of 4 HC in the presence of an irradiated allogeneic stromal cell layer. Moreover, the ability to generate these cells was increased when combinations of hematopoietic growth factors including stem cell factor and IL-3 were added. After 11-21 days of culture, the generation of colony-forming cells from CD34+Lin– 4-HC-treated cells was equivalent to that seen from untreated CD34+Lin– cells. Additional studies further identified the phenotype of these 4-HC-resistant CD34+Lin– precursors as CD38–, presumably reflective of their quiescent state. Thus, maximal stimulation of the growth of the most immature stem-cell-containing subpopulation of CD34+Lin– cells requires an as yet undefined interaction with marrow stroma in addition to known hematopoietic growth factors.

Summary

In-vivo studies have identified the human hematopoietic stem cell as a CD34+ cell that lacks a variety of antigens associated with T-cell, B-cell and myeloid cell differentiation. These cells also have the ability to resist treatment with 4-HC. In-vitro studies have demonstrated the ability of combinations of hematopoietic growth factors to stimulate the formation of colony-forming cells, but the 4-HC-resistant and presumably quiescent and least mature subset of these cells may require as yet undefined signal(s) from marrow stroma for optimal generation of the more differentiated progeny cells. Future identification of the factors required for optimal in-vitro generation of hematopoietic precursors, including perhaps the generation of increased numbers of stem cells, may allow us to use small samples of blood or marrow to prepare sufficient numbers of precursors suitable for reconstituting hematopoiesis in patients after myelosuppressive or myeloablative treatment.

References

1. Till JE, McCulloch EA. A direct measurement of the radiation sensitivity of normal mouse bone marrow cells. Radiat Res 1961;14:216-22.
2. Hodgson GS, Bradley TR, Radley JM. The organization of hemopoietic tissue as inferred from the effects of 5-fluorouracil. Exp Hematol 1982;10:26-35.

3. Bradley TR, Metcalf D. The growth of mouse bone marow cells in vitro. Aust J Exp Biol Med Sci 1966;44:287-99.
4. Pike BL, Robinson WA. Human bone marrow colony growth in agar-gel. J Cell Physiol 1970;76:77-84.
5. Stephenson JR, Axerad AA, McLeod DL, Shreeve MM. Induction of colonies of hemoglobin-synthesizing cells by erythropoietin in vitro. Proc Natl Acad Sci USA 1971;68:1542-6.
6. Tepperman AD, Curtis JE, McCulloch EA. Erythropietic colonies in cultures of human marrow. Blood 1974;44:659-69.
7. Clarke BJ, Housman D. Characterization of an erythroid precursor cell of high proliferative capacity in normal human peripheral blood. Proc Natl Acad Sci USA 1977;74:1105-9.
8. Fauser AA, Messner HA. Granuloerythropoietic colonies in human bone marrow, peripheral blood, and cord blood. Blood 1978;52:1243-8.
9. Keller G, Holmes W, Phillips RA. Clonal generation of multipotent and unipotent hemopoietic blast cell colonies in vitro. J Cell Physiol 1984;120:29-35.
10. Leary AG, Ogawa M. Blast cell colony assay for umbilical cord blood and adult bone marrow progenitors. Blood 1987;69:953-6.
11. Jones RJ, Wagner JE, Celano P, et al. Separation of pluripotent haematopoietic stem cells from spleen colony-forming cells. Nature 1990;347:188-9.
12. Civin CI, Strauss LC, Brovall C, et al. Antigenic analysis of hematopoiesis. III. A hematopoietic progenitor cell surface antigen defined by a monoclonal antibody raised against KG-1a cells. J Immunol 1984;133:157-65.
13. Tindle RW, Nichols RA, Chan L, et al. A novel monoclonal antibody BI-3C5 recognizes myeloblasts and non-B non-T lymphoblasts in acute leukaemias and CGL blast crises, and reacts with immature cells in normal bone marrow. Leuk Res 1985;9:1-9.
14. Katz FE, Tindle R, Sutherland DR, Greaves MF. Identification of a membrane glycoprotein associated with haemopoietic progenitor cells. Leuk Res 1985;9:191-8.
15. Andrews RG, Singer JW, Bernstein ID. Monoclonal antibody 12-8 recognizes a 115 kD molecule present on both unipotent and multipotent hematopoietic colony-forming cells and their precursors. Blood 1986;67:842-5.

16. Watt SM, Karhi K, Gatter K, et al. Distribution and epitope analysis of the cell membrane glycoprotein (HPCA-1) associated with human hemopoietic progenitor cells. Leukemia 1987;1:417-26.

17. Lansdorp PM, Sutherland HJ, Eaves CJ. Selective expression of CD45 isoforms on functional subpopulations of CD34+ hemopoietic cells from human bone marrow. J Exp Med 1990;172:363-6.

18. Peault B, Weissman IL, Baum C, et al. Lymphoid reconstitution of the human fetal thymus in SCID mice with CD34+ precursor cells. J Exp Med 1991;174:1283-6.

19. Baum CM, Weissman IL, Tsukamoto AS, et al. Isolation of a candidate human hematopoietic stem-cell population. Proc Natl Acad Sci USA 1992;89:2804-8.

20. Kyoizumi S, Baum CM, Kaneshima H, et al. Implantation and maintenance of functional human bone marrow in SCID-hu mice. Blood 1992;79:1704-11.

21. Srour EF, Zanjani ED, Brandt JE, et al. Sustained human hematopoiesis in sheep transplanted in utero during early gestation with fractionated adult human bone marrow cells. Blood 1992;79:1404-12.

22. Berenson RJ, Andrews RG, Bensinger WI, et al. CD34+ marrow cells engraft lethally irradiated baboons. J Clin Invest 1988;81:951-5.

23. Berenson RJ, Bensinger WI, Hill RS, et al. Engraftment after infusion of CD34+ marrow cells in patients with breast cancer and neuroblastoma. Blood 1991;77:1717-22.

24. Andrews RG, Bryant EM, Bartelmez SH, et al. CD34+ marrow cells, devoid of T and B lymphocytes, reconstitute stable lymphopoiesis and myelopoiesis in lethally irradiated allogeneic baboons. Blood 1992;80:1693-701.

25. Shpall EJ, Jones RB, Franklin W, et al. CD34 positive (+) marrow and/or peripheral blood progenitor cells (PBPCs) provide effective hematopoietic reconstitution of breast cancer patients following high-dose chemotherapy with autologous hematopoietic progenitor cell support (abstract). Blood 1992;80 (Suppl 1):24a.

26. Bernstein ID, Singer JW, Andrews RG, et al. Treatment of acute myeloid leukemia cells in vitro with a monoclonal antibody recognizing a myeloid differentiation antigen allows normal progenitor cells to be expressed. J Clin Invest 1987;79:1153-9.

27. Bernstein ID, Singer JW, Smith FO, et al. Differences in the frequency of normal and clonal precursor of colony-forming cells in CML and AML. Blood 1992;79:1811-6.
28. Robertson MJ, Soiffer RJ, Freedman AS, et al. Human bone marrow depleted of CD33-positive cells mediates delayed but durable reconstitution of hematopoiesis: Clinical trial of MY9 monoclonal antibody-purged autografts for the treatment of acute myeloid leukemia. Blood 1992;79:2229-36.
29. Kaizer H, Stuart RK, Brookmeyer R, et al. Autologous bone marrow transplantation in acute leukemia: A phase I study of in vitro treatment of marrow with 4-hydroperoxycyclophosphamide to purge tumor cells. Blood 1985;65:1504-10.
30. Yeager AM, Kaizer H, Santos GW, et al. Autologous bone marrow transplantation in patients with acute nonlymphocytic leukemia, using ex vivo marrow treatment with 4-hydroperoxycyclophosphamide. N Engl J Med 1986;315:141-7.
31. Martin PJ, Hansen JA, Buckner CD, et al. Effects of in vitro depletion of T cells in HLA-identical allogeneic marrow grafts. Blood 1985;66:664-72.
32. Ramsay N, LeBien T, Nesbit M, McGlave P, et al. Autologous bone marrow transplantation for patients with acute lymphoblastic leukemia in second or subsequent remission: Results of bone marrow treated with monoclonal antibodies BA-1, BA-2, and BA-3 plus complement. Blood 1985;66:508-13.
33. Ball ED, Mills LE, Coughlin CT, et al. Autologous bone marrow transplantation in acute myelogenous leukemia: In vitro treatment with myeloid cell-specific monoclonal antibodies. Blood 1986;68:1311-5.
34. Ferrero D, De Fabritiis P, Amadori S, et al. Autologous bone marrow transplantation in acute myeloid leukemia after in-vitro purging with an anti-lacto-N-fucopentaose III antibody and rabbit complement. Leuk Res 1987;11:265-72.
35. Verfaillie CM, Miller WJ, Boylan K, McGlave PB. Selection of benign primitive hematopoietic progenitors in chronic myelogenous leukemia on the basis of HLA-DR antigen expression. Blood 1992;79:1003-10.
36. Bernstein ID, Leary AG, Andrews RG, Ogawa M. Blast colony-forming cells and precursors of colony-forming cells detectable in long term marrow culture express the same phenotype (CD33– CD34+). Exp Hematol 1991;19:680-2.

37. Andrews RG, Singer JW, Bernstein ID. Precursors of colony-forming cells in humans can be distinguished from colony-forming cells based on expression of the CD33 and CD34 antigens and light scatter properties. J Exp Med 1989;169:1721-31.
38. Bernstein ID, Andrews RG, Zsebo KM. Recombinant human stem cell factor (SCF) enhances the formation of colonies by CD34+ and CD34+lin– cells, and the generation of colony-forming cell progeny from CD34+lin– cells cultured with IL-3, G-CSF, or GM-CSF. Blood 1991;77:2316-21.
39. Andrews RG, Singer JW, Bernstein ID. Human hematopoietic precursors in long-term culture: Single CD34+ cells that lack detectable T cell, B cell, and myeloid cell antigens produce multiple colony-forming cells when cultured with marrow stromal cells. J Exp Med 1990;172:355-8.
40. Rowley SD, Brashem-Stein C, Andrews R, Bernstein ID. Hematopoietic precursors resistant to treatment with 4-hydroperoxycyclophosphamide: Requirement for an interaction with marrow stroma in addition to hematopoietic growth factors for maximal generation of colony-forming activity. Blood 1993;82:60-5.
41. Sutherland HJ, Eaves CJ, Eaves AC, et al. Characterization and partial purification of human marrow cells capable of initiating long-term hematopoiesis in vitro. Blood 1989;74:1563-70.
42. Verfaillie C, Blakolmer K, McGlave P. Purified primitive human hematopoietic progenitor cells with long-term in vitro repopulating capacity adhere selectively to irradiated bone marrow stroma. J Exp Med 1990;172:509-20.
43. Briddell RA, Broudy VC, Bruno E, et al. Further phenotypic characterization and isolation of human hematopoietic progenitor cells using a monoclonal antibody to the c-kit receptor. Blood 1992;79:3159-67.
44. Terstappen LW, Huang S, Safford M, et al. Sequential generations of hematopoietic colonies derived from single non-lineage-committed CD34+CD38– progenitor cells. Blood 1991;77:1218-27.
45. Huang S, Terstappen LW. Formation of haematopoietic microenvironment and haematopoietic stem cells from single human bone marrow stem cells. Nature 1992;360:745-9.

Index